Touching Light

How to Free Your Fiber-Optic Fascia

Touching Light: How to Free Your Fiber-Optic Fascia

Copyright © 2015 Ronelle Wood

All rights reserved

No part of this publication may be reproduced, distributed, or transmitted in any form or by any means, including photocopying, recording, or other electronic or mechanical methods, without the prior written permission of the publisher, except in the case of brief quotations embodied in critical reviews and certain other noncommercial uses permitted by copyright law. For permission requests, write to "Attention: Permissions" at the address below.

Published and distributed by:
True Body Publishing
305 E. Matilija Street, Suite K
Ojai, CA 93023
ronelle@ohmsanctuary.com
facebook.com/fiberopticfascia?fref=ts
facebook.com/OHMSanctuary?fref=tsArtist/263894860420006

Contact the publisher for information on author interviews or speaking engagements.

First Edition

Printed in the United States of America

Edited by Sonia Nordenson
Cover concept by Rene Norman
Cover by John Hargrove of Evolved Designs
Author photo by Cecilia Ortiz
Printed by CreateSpace, an Amazon.com company
Available on Kindle and other devices

ISBN-13: 978-1517236625
ISBN-10: 1517236622

To the memory of my grandfather,
"Grampy"—Verlyn Devere Bond,
the youngest of twelve and a ray of light
whose photons course through me to this day.

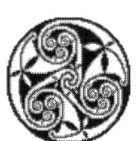

A photon checks into a hotel, and the bellhop asks if he can help him with his luggage. The photon replies, "No thanks, I'm traveling light."

Contents

Foreword by Gay Hendricks   1

Acknowledgments   3

Introduction   5

Chapter One: Doing What I Was Supposed to Do   9

Chapter Two: How I Met My Fascia   15

Chapter Three: The Worldwide Web Within You   23

Chapter Four: What Is Your "Net" Worth?   33

Chapter Five: When Fascia Is Injured   51

Chapter Six: Instinct Is Forever   57

Chapter Seven: MFR Is More Than Just Physical   65

Chapter Eight: Unwinding   81

Chapter Nine: "I'm Not Like That."   87

Chapter Ten: What a Practitioner Experiences   95

Chapter Eleven: Life in a Massage Mill   105

Chapter Twelve: Who's Healing Whom?   123

Chapter Thirteen: A Fascia Q&A   131

Chapter Fourteen: Fascia in the Future   147

Chapter Fifteen: Wrapping It Up   153

Epilogue   157

About the Author   161

Foreword

It is with great pleasure that I introduce you to the remarkable work and radiant being of Ronelle Wood. I've been blessed to know many great healers and teachers over my forty-five years in the field of transformation; Ronelle is right at the top of the list of masterful practitioners I've known.

I discovered Ronelle more than a year ago when two friends in the same week saw me limping along with my painful left knee and said, "You need to go see Ronelle Wood." I did, and my work with her has opened up a new world of ease and freedom in my body. My wife, Kathlyn, also works with Ronelle, so we have become a whole family of fascia-enthusiasts.

I admire many things about Ronelle and her work. First, she is absolutely and passionately committed to helping people feel great in their bodies. It is rare to be in the presence of someone so dedicated to the healing path she teaches. Second, the quality of her being and the space she creates invites deep exploration in a gentle, friendly way. Although the work is often intense, it is always as intense as you want it to be.

Ronelle's sensitivity is unparalleled in my experience. She is also blessed with the gifts of patience, compassion, and a wild sense of humor. The latter is, in my view, an essential quality for any true healer and masterful teacher to have.

I found Ronelle's explanation of the theoretical principles and technical information in the book to be illuminating. I'm not an expert in fascia or body mechanics, but I've had a professional interest in somatic transformation since I entered the field in 1968.

From that perspective, the focus on fascia and related concepts opened up a new dimension of knowledge for me. Specifically, awareness of the light and fiber-optic nature of fascia gave me an expanded sense of the importance of this area of our anatomy.

This book will certainly speak to professionals looking for significant innovations in the field of body-mind healing. However, I also recommend it to those of you who come to it for personal reasons, to seek relief from pain and a more loving relationship with your own body.

Ronelle's work reliably assists me in feeling a more spacious sense of ease as I move through the world. I urge you to experience directly what she and her trainees have to offer you.

I've often thought, in the midst of a session with Ronelle, that I'd like everyone in the world to be touched in such a loving, transformational way. Until that time, *Touching Light* is an excellent first step along the path.

Gay Hendricks, PhD
Author of *The Big Leap*

Acknowledgments

I thank the injuries and experiences that led me to seek healing, as well as the pivotal people who were catalysts in my awakening from illusion: my children, Genevieve and Alex; my dad; my brother, Edwin; Lifespring; John Barnes; and Alison Armstrong.

I am grateful for the unconditional love of my sister, Bonnie Jenkins, and my niece, Shauna Underwood.

I'm also grateful to have been quietly and peacefully alone with my mother, Carolee, as she passed from this life. It was an honor and a privilege to be chosen in that way and I promise that I will use the life she gave me to make a positive impact in this world.

I have undying appreciation for my beloved Joseph Aaron Cocke, whose love for me and passion for fascia make my life extraordinary.

In opening their lives to me and trusting me with their bodies, my clients and students continue to teach me and give to me.

I offer my heartfelt thanks to the scientists whose inquiry and persistence brought fascia into view—especially Dr. Jean-Claude Guimberteau.

I thank Lynne McTaggart for her compilation of research on consciousness.

I deeply appreciate my student and editor, Sonia Nordenson.

And my lifelong gratitude goes to Gay Hendricks, for his friendship, for trusting me with his psychedelic fascia, and for inspiring me to make the leap from my zone of excellence into my zone of genius—and that included writing this flippin' book.

Introduction

You have inside of you a cloak of gossamer connective tissue that surrounds and supports *everything* and functions like fiber optics. This tissue is called fascia.

For our purposes, the definition of *fascia* is: A sheet or band of fibrous tissue that envelopes, separates, or binds together muscles, organs, and other soft structures of the body—or a tissue occurring within such a sheet or band. The plural is *fasciae*, but in this book we'll use the word *fascia* as it's colloquially spoken, as a collective noun.

We now know that fascia is a web that connects everything in the body. It's like a body stocking, but one that also penetrates into the deep physical structures, surrounding everything inside us. The world's previous understanding came from studying fascia on cadavers. The dead connective tissue appeared to the naked eye to be something like cotton candy—dry and brittle.

Today, the true beauty of fascia can be seen in *living* color. In 2005 the French physician Jean-Claude Guimberteau, MD, used his fiber-optic surgical equipment to record and demonstrate what live fascia looks like.

He released a film called *Strolling Under the Skin* that, for the very first time, showed living connective tissue—magnified twenty-five times—so that we could see the tiny microtubules never before known to us.

Thanks to Dr. Guimberteau, we can now peer inside a human being and see that fascia is comprised of hollow, transparent, fluid-filled tubules that conduct light.

With Dr. Guimberteau's kind permission, I narrated a brief YouTube video of clips excerpted from *Strolling Under the Skin,* showing some of his amazing footage. It's titled *Living Fascia 25x Magnified (Narrated)*. In it, you can see for yourself what connective tissue looks like under magnification. Type the title into your search engine, or use your smart phone to read this QR code:

In their healthy state, the fascial fibers are very well hydrated, so that the strands remain individualized, running in the same direction as the muscles. When the fibers become dehydrated, they start to stick to each other.

Where fascia has been torn or cut, it repairs like plaid, layering itself every which way: up, down, crisscross, and diagonal, creating a scar. As it works to restore stability, it can even attach to nearby structures.

The fascia also thickens where the body is repeatedly overused (such as when we're texting, driving, sitting, etc.) or where there are patterns of holding (tight throat, hunched shoulders, clenched buttocks), forming bundles much like unstirred spaghetti in a pot of boiling water. If left unstretched, those bundles of fascia can ossify (i.e., turn to bone).

In her book *The Field: The Quest for the Secret Force of the Universe*, Lynne McTaggart cites Karl H. Pribram, Kunio Yasue, Stuart Hameroff, and Scott Hagan, whose research brought them to the theory that there is a system of "light pipes" that form "the Internet of the body" and share information through photons. These light pipes account for the speed at which information travels throughout the body—much faster than nerve impulses can carry electric signals.

With the benefit of this theory, I can now better explain the fascinating changes I've seen happen for clients in my twelve-year practice of *myofascial release* or MFR.

This form of bodywork, in which I was trained by founder John Barnes, PT, treats the connective tissue by using gentle traction and compression on the skin, without oil.

This book is about what I've learned so far regarding the amazing gossamer web of fascia within us, and it's about my own experiences in alleviating the pain of fascial restriction through giving, receiving, and teaching myofascial release.

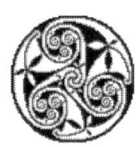

Chapter One
Doing What I Was Supposed to Do

I touch people for a living. I wasn't supposed to be doing this; I didn't set out to. I wasn't raised to. I was supposed to be a Seventh Day Adventist, a doctor's wife, a mother, and a speech pathologist.

I started out doing what I was "supposed to do"—what my parents and the church expected of me. It involved hard work, dedication, perseverance, and a lot of studying far into the night, all in order to be prepared, to be ready to accomplish and achieve.

Eventually I climbed to the top of my mountain of academic achievement, and then I started down the other side and made my way into the working world.

The path I'd traveled to get to this point had included countless hours spent studying language development, articulation, dysfluency, aphasia, statistics. I learned and retained a lot of interesting tidbits that I remember to this day: e.g., comprehension comes before expression, and nouns emerge first and verbs are second.

Phonetic symbols can be used to represent all of the sounds in our language. With cool little symbols like æ, ŋ, and ʃ, I had learned to exactly transcribe anybody's talking pattern. The stuttering caused by difficulties with speech fluency fascinated me. I'd studied neuroscience with its axons, dendrites, synapses, and neurotransmitters, had learned the areas of the brain and what they were known to govern. I understood audiology, hearing loss, and auditory processing disorders. I'd studied how a stroke can result in aphasia, speech impairment, or cognitive impairment.

I had been thoroughly tested to ensure that I knew all the treatment approaches for each speech disorder. I sometimes felt buried under a pile of lesson plans and SOAP notes. (SOAP—an acronym for subjective, objective, assessment, and plan—is a method of documentation employed by healthcare providers to write out notes in a patient's chart.) Through inner city schools, I'd earned a hard-won teaching credential.

As my comprehensive exams approached, I can remember having the most severe anxiety of my life to that point. A tremendous amount of struggle had gone into obtaining this education while working to pay for it, and everything was riding on the results of those exams.

Questions swirled in my head. *Will this all be for naught? How many ways do I have to prove I'm worthy of graduating? And then prove that I'm worthy of being hired somewhere?*

I survived the rigors of graduate school and marched out into the world, armed with my Master of Science degree in Speech/Language Pathology from California State University, Sacramento.

I landed my first job at a head trauma clinic, where I specialized in treating speech and cognitive disorders resulting from brain injury. My heart ached for those patients, who included young male survivors of accidents, a woman who at twenty-one had had a brain aneurysm burst, and geriatric patients who had fallen and incurred head injuries.

My next job was as an itinerant speech pathologist. I drove from homes to schools to other schools to homes again, carrying out the directives of a boss who had secured contracts and insurance payments and who paid me one quarter of the fee she collected for the work I did.

I worried all the time that I was not able to really help. Conversations with my boss included exchanges like this:

Me: "The stroke patient I've been seeing for three weeks has not made any measureable progress, and he's now expressing discouragement."

Her: "Well, the insurance company has authorized twelve visits, so you just need to keep seeing him."

In my fourth year of practice, I began to experience physical symptoms: aches and pains in my back, arms, and legs.

My solution was to schedule a weekly massage, and I looked forward to that time more than anything else all week.

My doctor husband didn't hold the practice of massage therapy in high regard. His church-taught idea of "massage" was probably more along the lines of "massage parlor." But I would escape to my appointments and come home feeling better. I didn't care if he thought I was being self-indulgent, it helped me to cope.

I was sitting *all the time*, often in tiny chairs, and walking in high heels. When the masseuse worked on my hips, back, and feet, it was absolute heaven.

One day I blurted to her, "You must have the best job in the world, because you know that, right now, this minute, you're making someone feel better."

I didn't realize that this was a person who was less limited in her thinking—someone who saw choice and possibilities everywhere. Someone who, obviously, didn't share my worldview, and in her naïveté suggested that I get my massage therapy license. How ridiculous was that?

I responded by saying, "I spent seven years in college to do what I do for a living. I have two small children. I have a job and responsibilities. I couldn't do that."

To which she responded, "I'll watch your kids for you." How ridiculous that she thought it could be that easy.

Three months later I had my massage therapy license from the Santa Barbara School of Massage. With the full disapproval of my children's father, I began dabbling in touching people. Of course, it was just a hobby, only a side interest.

I loved it.

After a year of having one foot in speech pathology and the other in massage therapy, I finally made the leap toward what I loved. I have never once regretted it. I don't look back with sadness at having left behind all the driving, the paperwork, the SOAP notes, the grappling with insurance companies over getting paid, and all of the stress and tension I brought on myself by doing a job that I didn't love.

I could not have known then where my choice at this fork in the road was going to lead me. I had no clue that I was choosing to follow a transformational path. I didn't realize how much my clients would affect me. I wasn't aware of how much fulfillment was yet to be discovered in my life.

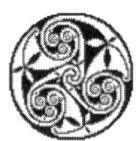

Chapter Two
How I Met My Fascia

After I'd practiced massage therapy for eight years, the woman with whom I shared a business began to encourage me to look into something called the John F. Barnes Myofascial Release Approach®. My office partner had taken one of John Barnes's seminars, and had really loved it.

She tried a little bit of it on me, and I didn't get it. I thought the name of the treatment was ugly, and I was less than amused. I had seen it advertised to an annoying degree in my monthly *Massage & Bodywork* magazine. I was convinced that this was just one more fellow trying to make a name for himself by doing what I already knew how to do, but with some trademark snake-oil type of twist that he could put his name on and claim fame for having invented.

Yet my business partner wouldn't let it go. She prompted and prodded and pushed and cajoled. Or at least that's what it felt like. (In reality, she quietly mentioned it, and probably only a couple of times a year.)

After two years, she was finally able to move this stubborn woman who already knew it all toward something new. I chose the closest, cheapest, shortest seminar they had to offer: "The Fascial Pelvis," taught by a woman named Tina. I seriously doubted that this woman could teach me anything of value. This myofascial release work was supposed to be the brainchild of John F. Barnes, PT. So where was *he*?

I sat in the back row with my arms crossed, waiting for Tina to show me something I didn't know. She bored me with a lecture and slides. I squirmed in my seat. *Isn't this just great, sitting again.*

When it came time for the demonstration phase, Tina asked for volunteers. A woman in perfect physical shape hopped up and—just like that—began stripping down to her underwear as she made her way to the front of the conference room and got on the demo table. I told myself she was obviously a "plant" in the audience.

Tina had the woman lie face up so that she could demonstrate a "sacral hold." Lying on her back with her knees bent and feet on the table, the volunteer raised her hips as Tina reached under her, through the woman's legs, and placed her palm on the lowest part of the volunteer's spine, the sacrum. Then the woman lowered her hips, straightened her legs, and just lay there while Tina's palm tractioned slightly toward the woman's feet.

The woman on the table moaned and writhed a little bit, and I thought, *She's faking it. Anybody could do that. These California people* . . .

By this point in the seminar, the woman sitting next to me had begun to "stick out." I noticed (and judged) that she asked too many questions, gave too many anecdotal stories, and was clearly all up in her ego. I made a mental note that, when it was time to work on each other in pairs, I would make sure not to get paired up with her.

So, in the way of this great comical universe, I got paired with her. We were going to practice this same sacral hold. I knew that I could probably provide her with some therapeutic effect. I was doubtful that anything she did would be helpful to me.

She went first. She moaned a little, moved a little. I was unimpressed.

Then it was my turn. To have someone cradle the triangular bone at the base of your spine by reaching between your legs when you're lying face up is essentially having someone invade your personal space *big time*.

As I lay there on my back, staring at the ceiling with the woman's hand on my sacrum, I began to realize how angry I was feeling. I closed my eyes and attempted to endure this indignity till it was over.

I was surprised to feel a finger touch my chin. It was Tina the instructor. She whispered in my ear, "Let that sound out."

I realized that my chin was wiggling with the effort that it took to hold in the frustration I was feeling. So I gently parted my lips and let out the tiniest little squeak— in retrospect, quite pitiful.

17

The instructor retrieved a pillow and laid it in my arms, telling me that it was okay to let that sound out into the pillow. I was thinking, Jack Nicholson style, *You can't HANDLE that sound.*

I don't know what made me take the chance. It seemed that an avalanche of emotion, a lifetime of being polite and appropriate and fitting in and not rocking the boat, was about to burst its dam. A very strong feeling of *Screw it—you asked for it!* came over me, and I opened my mouth, letting out the most bloodcurdling scream of my life. This was followed by an audible and physical expression of all the anger, holding, inhibition, and suppression that I had accrued in a lifetime of being a good girl.

My internal monitor/censor/editor was in a panic. The voice in my head was shouting, *All the other therapists in this room could have been potential referral sources! That's over now. You've done it. You're that girl! You're out of control. You're crazy, just like your mother!*

After a period of time that involved some flailing about of my limbs and a huge amount of noise and tears, I began to hear people whispering:

"We need to get back to class."

"Find her a blanket."

"This shaking she's doing is accomplishing a lot."

And the last whisper: "Ronelle, when you feel ready, you can come back to your seat."

I peeked through my eyelids, expecting to see horrified, worried faces staring down at me. All I saw were reassuring smiles, and no one appeared the least bit frightened.

I tried with all my might to get it together as fast as I could. Although I wasn't cold, I was shaking like a leaf. I felt embarrassed, confused, and completely undone. This was the kind of "crazy" I had tried a lifetime not to be, and here I was being it in front of colleagues. *I guess I could always go back to speech pathology*, I thought.

I eventually made it out from under the blanket and up off the table. I tiptoed to the bathroom, trying not to interrupt the lecture that had been resumed.

When I got to the bathroom and looked in the mirror, I saw little red petechiae around my eyes—something I hadn't seen since I gave birth to my second child.

That was the moment when I knew that all of the physical and emotional expression from the day I checked into a hospital three thousand miles from home, with no photo I.D. and no insurance card, a twenty-month-old toddler, and a husband who was about to strand me there for three months, had been held inside me for the last ten years.

Pregnant and Far from Home

In 1992, I was great with child. My second.

According to the University of North Carolina's specialized study using an intra-vaginal ultrasound wand, the size of my baby indicated that my own calculated due date of May 15 was incorrect. The doctors informed me that I should expect to deliver sometime in the beginning of June.

My husband and I had negotiated a truce. In spite of my strong desire to return home to California, I had agreed to deliver our first child in North Carolina. It had now been two years, and he had realized, "If mama ain't happy, ain't nobody happy." So in April we'd gone on a job interview to the Santa Barbara Medical Foundation Clinic. The job would be at a satellite clinic in Santa Maria, 70 miles to the north. I thought, *How different could that be?*

We found out. The difference, to me, was huge. Whereas Santa Barbara has a temperate climate and miles of beautiful beaches attracting tourists and the very wealthy from Los Angeles, Santa Maria is an agricultural town built on the strawberry industry . . . because strawberries love overcast skies and cooler temperatures. The nearest beach—a short stretch of rocky shore pounded by merciless wind and unrelenting surf—is thirteen miles away.

But I didn't care. I was gung ho to move back to California, wherever it was.

We were invited back for a second interview. I bundled up the many trappings that go with having a 20-month-old and waddled through airports with my daughter till we arrived in Sacramento, there to spend time with my sister before my husband flew out to join us for the interview.

On the day of the interview, I drove a rental car to the Sacramento airport. As I attempted to return the car, I realized my wallet was missing. I turned the car inside out and still couldn't find it. Time was passing, my tension was mounting, and I didn't want to miss the flight, so I returned the rental car, wedged myself and my baby girl into a puddle jumper, and flew to Santa Maria.

Reservations had been made for us to stay at the Santa Maria Inn. The loss of my wallet was an ever-present tension in the back of my mind, and caused a minor snag when I checked in. But luckily the kind folks from the Santa Barbara Medical Foundation Clinic were willing to vouch for me by telephone.

As I arrived in our room, I was holding my daughter over my big belly. Kneeling on the bed to lay her down, I felt an immediate sharp pain. I stood up, and saw that I had knelt on a bee, its stinger now embedded in my knee. What were the odds?

But as my focus shifted I realized that the room was full of bees. We were on the ground floor in an older wing of the inn, which boasted a beautiful rose garden just outside. Hence the swarm of wildlife that had made its way indoors.

We moved to a higher floor in a newer end of the hotel. My knee was sore, but I was going to be just fine.

That night at 11 p.m. (2 a.m. Eastern time), my husband arrived, and that night I began feeling some very regular contractions . . . At 1 a.m. on May 16, three thousand miles from home and my OB/GYN, we called a taxi and asked the driver to take us, along with our toddler daughter, to a hospital. He asked, "Which one?" as if we would know.

The hospital we chose naturally asked for my identification and health insurance card. Somehow we found our way through the delivery of a healthy baby boy at 8:30 the next morning. Later I caught a glimpse of myself in a mirror and saw little red petechia around my eyes, indicating tiny burst blood vessels from the exertion of pushing my baby boy into this world.

It was interview day. The doctors saw their way clear to hire my husband in spite of the wacky circumstances. All seemed to be well, with the exception of a few complications that needed to be handled.

First, my husband had to return to North Carolina to finish out the last three months of his contract there. Second, we didn't have a place to live.

I flew back up to Sacramento, and in those first few weeks my sister helped with the new baby and my toddler daughter. I was able to find a furnished condo in Santa Maria, and my sister drove us there and helped us move in, although her job as CFO of Mercy Hospitals required her to return rather quickly.

There in Santa Maria, I began a solitary journey of caring for my new baby, my little girl, and myself. I didn't have time to let down; I had to power on. And so I did.

Ten years later, as I stared at my reflection in the mirror and saw those red petechiae around my eyes, I made the connection. My body was telling on me, and it had so much to say.

I realized that I was now ready to learn more about this myofascial release business.

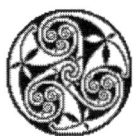

Chapter Three
The Worldwide Web Within You

Many people read or hear the word *fascia* and imagine that it has something to do with a spa treatment for your face or an oppressive, dictatorial government. But, with education and repetition, the word is now coming into more widespread use.

The term *fascia* is becoming a household word, for books and research on the topic abound. Some of the texts are so full of heavy scientific language describing the components, chemistry, function, and physiology of fascia that it can be confusing and hard to translate.

My aim is to share my experience as a myofascial release therapist and explain how fascia affects us in everyday life.

Knowing about fascia will give you a brand new view of your body. You'll be able to let go of the notion that your physical self is something beyond your understanding, something disconnected into separate pieces that can be removed and replaced without consequence. And you'll no longer hold the perception that your body is a misbehaving slave needing to be punished into submission.

Physical Fiber Optics

Fiber optics, the thin, transparent fibers of glass or plastic now used in thousands of diverse scientific and commercial settings, transmit electromagnetic information from one place to another by conducting pulses of light through lengths of optical fibers.

In one medical application, a bundle of such fibers is used in an instrument designed to view body cavities. It took one to photograph one. That is, as you read in the introduction, thanks to Jean-Claude Guimberteau, fiber-optic cameras can now be used to capture on film the fiber-optic nature of human fascia.

Prior to Dr. Guimberteau's film *Strolling Under the Skin*, myofascial release therapists all over the world could only speculate about the properties of the connective tissue they were working with. Many tried to issue descriptions.

Anatomist Gil Hedley studied fascia on cadavers and, in a popular YouTube video that caused quite a stir in the communities that study fascia, made the assertion that fascia was "fuzz" that grew inside the body at night.

Unfortunately, because of Hedley filming dead connective tissue and calling it fuzz, those wanting to learn about fascia were led far afield from what *living* fascia actually looks like, as well as the functions that it serves.

Science has known of the body's light-bearing quality since 1923, when the Russian biologist and medical scientist Alexander Gurwitsch first detected the phenomenon of the biophoton, or radiant emittance in the ultraviolet spectrum, of biological tissues of the human body.

In her book *The Field*, Lynne McTaggart explains how researchers pursuing for decades an understanding of the function and origin of human consciousness reached the conclusion that photons are transmitted through "light pipes" in the body.

McTaggart writes: "This would provide an explanation for the instantaneous operation of our brains, which occurs at between one ten-thousandth and one-thousandth of a second, requiring that information be transmitted at one hundred to one thousand meters per second—a speed that exceeds the capabilities of any known connections between axons or dendrites in neurons." In other words, "light pipe" information is transmitted much faster than the speed at which nerve impulses travel.

This Book Goes Beyond Theory

This account of my experience as an MFR practitioner will tell you why fascia has been the missing link in our understanding of human health, disease, fitness, wellness, energy, and emotion.

On the topic of fascia, it will point out the difference between the theoretical and the actual. As you read, you'll remember. Your body will begin to offer you memories of past accidents, injuries, and other traumas.

A client on my treatment table once murmured through the face cradle, "This is exactly what I have never known I always wanted." That phrase perfectly captures the feeling and substance of myofascial release.

If what you read in these pages leads you to find the healing you've been seeking, then I'll have achieved one main purpose of this book. Yet I have in mind an even greater purpose. The world needs more people who do this work, so if you're someone who desires to effectively help others heal, avoid surgery, and maintain vibrant health, I hope to inspire *you* to become an MFR practitioner.

Body therapists have been divided into two categories: manual and movement. Manual therapists are those who touch your body while you passively receive. Movement therapists are those who teach you how to move your body to best effect.

In my practice, I combine:

- An understanding of the light-conducting nature of fascia
- The manual treatment of myofascial release
- Movement instruction to correct dysfunctional body mechanics
- A maintenance program of classes to help clients sustain optimal alignment following treatment

The unique protocol of my True Body™ work came about through my own search for healing. In this book I describe some of the physical traumas of my own life experience, and how I found my way out of their debilitating residual effects. I can now appreciate the past negative events of my life, for they led to my understanding of the function of fascia and how to walk every day to support optimal alignment. In my search for healing, I not only found what worked; I also found my gift.

What We Need to Know About Fascia

Surgeons have been taught that fascia is like packing material, and they still see it as "the stuff in the way" when they're trying to cut through a body.

If you can ever bring yourself to watch one of the millions of surgeries viewable on YouTube, one of the first things you'll see, after the initial incision, is the physician using his scalpel to sheer as many layers of fascia as he can, as fast as he can, to expose the anatomical target he's after.

To see an example of this, if you have a strong stomach you can do a YouTube search for "Fascia Cut During Surgery" or scan this QR code:

I wish that surgeons knew the long-term effects this scalpel slashing has on a patient's fascia. When the cut tissue heals, the biological response is to make the area stronger than it was before. The repairing fibers don't lie in the same direction as the muscle, but are diagonal and crisscrossed. As they work to stabilize the wound, they may surround and adhere to other structures in the vicinity.

As the fascia makes its repairs, it thickens and becomes less flexible, causing the surrounding tissue to be inhibited in its normal range of motion as well. The incision from a Caesarean section, for one common example, can result in a scar that gradually surrounds and attaches to the intestinal tract, the uterus, and the ovaries, causing pain, poor circulation, and limited mobility.

The scar begins to strangle the natural peristalsis of the intestines or the healthy range of motion and lymphatic and circulatory flow in the abdomen and hips. Years later, this same woman might present with abdominal pain, and might be evaluated for Crohn's disease, irritable bowel syndrome, or pelvic floor disorder when what's actually going on is an overgrowth of scar tissue from a procedure performed years ago.

Unfortunately, the medical profession has not yet caught up with this information, and patients are still being told that an accident or surgery that happened years ago couldn't possibly be related to the pain, complications, and limited range of motion they are experiencing today. Until they update their understanding of the fascia, doctors can't prepare patients with this knowledge before a surgery and can't routinely prescribe myofascial release as a necessary post-surgical treatment.

If they were to do that, such treatment would increase circulation, shorten recovery time, decrease the formation of adhesions, hasten the return to a normal range of motion, and reduce pain and the need for long-term pain medication.

My Gallbladder Surgery

When I was married, my doctor husband told me about some of the acronyms and alliterative lists that physicians use for diagnoses or shorthand communication between colleagues. For instance, they might say, "I've got a real GOMER in Room 2."

"GOMER" is an acronym for "Get out of my emergency room." This might refer to someone who was a frequent visitor with trivial complaints, or a "train wreck" with an unhealthy lifestyle who hadn't followed his doctor's orders and came in to the ER on a weekend to be fixed.

Another acronym was "FLK"—their way of communicating to one another that they were seeing a child who, based on the child's physical appearance, possibly had birth defects. Wide-set eyes, low-set ears, short fingers, a small chin, or a protruding tongue, among other physical traits, could be indications of Down syndrome, fetal alcohol syndrome, and other birth defects. The acronym stood for "funny looking kid," and I always considered its use to be a result of the jading effects of doctors' overexposure to human suffering.

One alliterative list my husband told me about was one that I never forgot: female, fat, flatulent, and forty. This list helped them to diagnose a possible gallbladder issue.

In my late thirties, I was a stay-at-home mom with two children and two stepchildren. The boys were nine and ten, and the girls eleven and fourteen. I was functioning at maximum capacity in the areas of patience, energy, and marital relationship. That is to say, I was tired and unfulfilled.

I understand only in retrospect that I was looking for a break.

I took my symptoms to a doctor, who referred me to a surgeon. And, as happens when you ask a surgeon what she thinks, surgery was recommended. I tried to pin her down as to exactly what the ultrasound showed that made her suggest surgery. She said, "It was slightly murky, no visible stones; we could take a wait-and-see approach. It might resolve, or you might need to have it removed later on if your symptoms worsen."

My prior experiences of being hospitalized, to get my tonsils removed when I was four and for mastitis when I was a nursing mother, had involved getting lots of rest and attention. This made the surgeon's suggestion seem appealing, so I gave my consent.

The surgeon had described how she would perform the surgery using laparoscopic tools through my navel. Yet I awoke from the surgery to see a significant one-inch incision from my navel downward and two incisions beneath the ribs on my right side.

Recovery was horrible. Through the next three months, I experienced levels of pain that made me wish death would come. I remember having the clear thought, *If this is what the rest of my life is going to feel like, it's not worth it.* Yet I had no idea what far-reaching effects that small procedure would have on my body for the rest of my life.

I later saw, in X-rays a chiropractor took of my back, the bright white outlines of two plastic clips still inside me—standard procedure, I learned. Worse still, the surgeon had inserted a laparoscopic tool into my belly button and followed a path toward my gallbladder with no regard for the intervening connective tissue. Those clips inside me, and the scarring and myofascial effect of that laparoscopic procedure, affect my alignment and digestion to this day.

When the fascia surrounding the intestines is healthy, the pathways are wide open and digestion flows smoothly. When the fascia clamps down and scarring occurs, it narrows areas of the intestines and inhibits smooth digestion.

If patients who are several or many years post-surgery don't know the cause of their discomfort, they may go in search of other explanations and end up on laxatives, antacids, anti-inflammatory drugs, or pain medications.

That experience gave me firsthand awareness that cutting into a person is no small thing. The effects can be far-reaching and long-lasting. I feel deeply grateful for the myofascial release I've received for this issue, and thankful that I didn't waste a lot of time trying to chase an elusive diagnosis for why I felt so twisted up internally.

Doctors of the Future

Thomas Edison once said: "The doctor of the future will give no medicine but will interest his patients in the care of the human frame, in diet, and in the cause and prevention of disease."

In the future, I believe it will become standard protocol for physicians to prescribe MFR following surgery. My experience was that it had fully as much value in my healing process as did physical therapy. When more clinical trials have been conducted and reliable data collected, the results will verify what we see and what our clients report.

Myofascial release creates better outcomes, as measured by fewer complaints of pain, fewer complications following surgery, and reductions in the number of post-surgical office visits. It restores or improves range of motion and results in an earlier return to normal function.

In fact, the medical system already acknowledges the efficacy of this treatment. Myofascial pain syndrome is internationally classified as a disease (ICD-9 729.1), and in the United States myofascial release has its own national treatment classification code (CPT 97140). Patients in the U.S. can request a prescription for this treatment from their doctor, and medical insurance covers a percentage of the cost.

Chapter Four
What Is Your "Net" Worth?

On car trips, my dad would get fed up with the three kids in the back seat tittering, bickering, and being silly, and he'd reach back while he was driving and find the first knee he could grab. He'd squeeze his thumb and fingers on either side of that knee with all his might, till the one being suppressed was subdued.

But knowing that we weren't supposed to make any noise only made it worse. So we'd ride for a few more miles inciting each other and suppressing our laughter, trying not to look at each other, but we weren't usually successful. A giggle would burst its dam, causing the other two siblings to explode as well. As a result, I developed some mighty tight holding patterns in my knees that were mysteriously connected to tightness in my throat.

The quality of our internal web of fascia depends on a number of factors. As that childhood memory of mine illustrates, we humans start from an early age to form fascial holding patterns according to how we're taught to behave. As we learn to exert voluntary control over our movements, these holding patterns take over and we become unconscious of them. Our fascia thickens according to the physical movements we most often repeat—think of the amount of time children spend bent into classroom chairs during the most critical years of their physical growth.

Add to that the moments of fear (whether or not an injury occurred) when the body tightened. Pile on a few common spills off a bicycle, tumbles down a staircase, or falls from a tree, fence, or trampoline, and you realize that, gravity being what it is, a body experiences countless moments of fascial clenching.

Finally we add any actual rending of the tissue, whether from intentional surgery or unintentional scrapes, cuts, or tears. We become a puzzle of "trick" knees, tight places, "weak" ankles, a "bad" shoulder, areas that "pull," a back that "goes out," and areas of limited range of motion, to name just a few puzzle pieces.

We need all the room we can get in our fascial web. Yet, with each experience of clenching that I've just described, we lose circulation into the farthest reaches of our body and find ourselves having less ease of movement.

Allow me to shed more light on just how we're put together, so that you can exert more conscious choice about your "worldwide web within."

Fascial Structure

Fascia is primarily composed of the load-bearing structural proteins collagen and elastin. This means that, thanks to the collagen, your connective tissue has the ability to both stiffen and melt, and that, because of the elastin, it can both contract and stretch.

To give you a picture of how your body is put together in terms of fascia, imagine peeling an orange, as demonstrated in the video you'll find by searching YouTube for "Fascia Orange Analogy" or scanning this QR code:

Once you've removed the peel, you still have a round ball in your hand. It's the orange's white "connective tissue"—its pith—that keeps the shape of the orange.

You are like that. Under your skin, there's a superficial layer of fascia that surrounds everything and maintains your shape. Because of this connective tissue, all of your internal workings wouldn't just fall down around your ankles if your skin were gone.

Taking this analogy further, you can separate each section of an orange from the rest, because each has its own surrounding container. You're like that as well. Every individual organ and muscle inside of you is surrounded by its own fascial layer.

Let's go another layer deeper. You can open an orange slice and find that each little piece of pulp has *its* own surrounding layer of tissue. You are also like that. Human fascia surrounds your every muscle spindle and organelle, all the way down to each and every bone.

And bone is just mineralized fascia. This explains why, while we're working on the surface of your skin, you might sometimes feel the pull of the traction so deeply that the sensation seems to wrap down around your bones.

Because the fascia forms a web, and connects everything to everything, you can be receiving myofascial release on your neck and feel a sensation in your foot. It often happens that, when I'm working somewhere on a client's upper body, that person will reach up to scratch her nose—always my opportunity to point out that this is not random happenstance but information about where the fascial patterns are tight and pulling.

Remembering the John Barnes adage *Treat the symptom; look elsewhere for the cause*, I let the itchy nose guide me to the connection between, say, her shoulder and her face—where I will also work. Itchiness always serves as a clue that will help me solve the fascial-restriction puzzle.

Each little fiber communicates with every other little fiber. With this understanding of the structure of the fascial system, you can see why the ancient Chinese practice of acupuncture developed the concept of the energetic lines called meridians.

Meridian lines follow predictable paths, connect all areas of the body, and can become blocked. The fascial fibers are the anatomical structure that the meridians follow.

The fascial layers also follow predictable pathways that can be traced throughout the body. Thomas Myers provides illustrations of these patterns in his book *Anatomy Trains: Myofascial Meridians for Manual and Movement Therapists*.

In performing dissection on cadavers, fascia researchers have recently discovered that using the scalpel horizontally, instead of vertically, allows for layers of fascial planes that surround muscle groups to be lifted like tectonic plates or the layers of a croissant.

A network of fascial fibers called the *back line* begins at the bottom of the feet, goes up the entire back side of the body, up the neck, over the skull and ends at the arches of the eyebrows. Other networks follow a *front line*, a *lateral line*, and a *spiral line* as well.

In addition, sheets of fascia bisect the body from front to back in the same anatomical locations assigned to the chakras of Eastern philosophies. These transverse planes of connective tissue can be found in the areas of the pelvic floor, the hips, the diaphragm, the chest, the throat, and the eyes. To see a visual representation of these planes, go to www.ohmsanctuary.massagetherapy.com/myofascial-release or scan this QR code:

Fight, Flight, or Freeze

As we've established, fascia is a container, a connector, and a supporter. It is also a protector. With its two thousand pounds of tensile strength, it can resist a tremendous amount of force. This can make you incredibly strong when you're afraid.

In the body's involuntary freeze response to fear or pain, the fascia functions by contracting. During a fight-or-flight situation, every fascial fiber reacts protectively by clamping down. The purpose is to squeeze the blood vessels and nerves embedded in the fat and fascia, in order to inhibit pain and excessive bleeding. If you're in danger and need to fight or flee, this autonomic reaction of the sympathetic nervous system serves to keep you numb and lessen your chance of bleeding to death.

When you allow your body a fight-or-flight reaction following a fearful event—that is, when you let yourself kick or yell or punch or shake or run—your parasympathetic nervous system can then kick in with a rest-and-restore response.

When you voluntarily suppress those natural reactions, you enlist your fascia to carry out the inhibition, which it does by clamping down. In this case, you've given your parasympathetic system nothing to respond to, and it doesn't kick in.

Nuh-Uh

In certain times of stress and duress, we try to hide our animal nature. We tell our body, *Not now*.

This temporary fix, if left uninterrupted, eventually becomes an ingrained and unconscious holding pattern. Have you ever found yourself in a situation that was just too much for you to handle? For such occasions, we humans have an automatic survival technique known as denial.

Your patterning instantaneously determines that the consequences of an honest reaction to adrenaline would be *way* worse than just telling your body *Not now*. So a lightening-speed physical response inhibits your reaction.

From the time we're small, our parents begin socialization training to help us become acceptable in society. They admonish us to "Please sit down," "Please be quiet," and "Please hold still." And this is so hard for us at first. We have to be reminded over and over, because there's so much to learn and everything inside us is telling us to move and explore.

Slowly, our fascia takes over the job. We develop an efficient background program, like the operating system on a computer. The holding program inhibits our body to keep us "appropriate," and we're not usually consciously aware of it.

We learned to exert holding in the throat so that we wouldn't talk too loudly, say rude things, or tell family secrets. Most of us can recall a hand placed over our mouth, or a gasp and a consequence from a grownup, when we said out loud something that we were thinking, like, "Why does the skin under your chin hang down and wiggle when you talk?"

Our arms develop their own holding pattern, so that we don't reach out to slap someone or steal other kids' toys. And we all have holding in the belly, buttocks, and legs, acquired so that we don't kick people and run away laughing.

When we're young, we have a lot of opportunity to jump around, move in goofy ways, and discharge all that holding energy.

I get a kick out of watching children waiting while their mom chats with someone in the grocery store or at school pickup time. Little ones are completely uninhibited as they spin, flap their hands, play with their feet, roll on the ground, and otherwise take every opportunity to engage in movements that interrupt holding patterns.

Parents hope that, with age, their children will learn dignity. And, usually, the older we get the more appropriately we behave. On a daily basis, we become less and less likely to let our body jump around, move in goofy ways, or appear to be silly or out of control.

As a consequence, though, the body becomes progressively tighter and less flexible. There are so many instances in which we don't allow our body to move that it becomes, in effect, a storage house of experiences in the form of adrenaline, lactic acid, and uric acid—trapped against muscles by the fascial sleeves surrounding it. There it marinates and becomes sticky and gummy, causing restriction and inflexibility.

Every time you tell your body *Not now*, you hold *in* something that wanted to come *out*. There needs to be a time set aside for allowing your body to follow its natural unwinding movement. A time when you can tell your body, *Okay . . . now*.

"Oh, Yeah—I Had My Spleen Removed"

The ways that physical denial shows up in the body can be astounding. When I see someone for treatment for the first time, I ask about accidents and surgeries. These have significant effects on the fascia, and I want to get a brief overall view of what a given body has been through, up to that point, in its physical experience on Earth.

After an interview and the thorough review of a lifetime of movement that might include an assault, a tummy tuck, a car accident, breast augmentation, skateboarding into a wall, tumbles from trees, fences, horses, or bicycles, or the gamut of surgeries from a tonsillectomy to a hip replacement, we begin treatment.

I begin touching the client's skin and applying compression and traction, and often it isn't until after he has been on the treatment table for awhile and brought his attention back into his body that a memory is released to him that had been completely hidden from his current awareness. As you can gather from the following actual statements of clients, some astounding information is revealed.

"I forgot to tell you, I had my spleen removed."

"I have a titanium plate in my head."

"I fell off the back of a car bumper while my friend was driving. I hit my head, but arranged my hair to cover the huge bump so I wouldn't get in trouble with my parents."

"I had a mastectomy, and they used my stomach muscle as a flap for reconstruction."

"I lost a lot of weight when I was young, and had the excess skin surgically removed from all over my body."

"When I was born, my parents lived in a castle in Germany with thick walls of stone. Their doctor told them to leave me in the pram at one end of the castle to cry it out, so they wouldn't be tempted to comfort me when I was colicky."

Given my own experiences in life (which long lay buried and denied, deep in my tissues, making me feel like I might let loose one day, lose my sanity, and never get it back), I realize that only the tip of an iceberg of trauma might be revealed in this way. The gift of my own past traumatic experiences is that I am not surprised by what is revealed.

Everyone has fascia that has been constricted around muscle for years, holding encapsulated cocktails of chemistry—the lactic acid, uric acid, and adrenaline that are byproducts of fear.

Only when there is both an invitation from the outside to explore deeper (as I place my hands on your skin), and permission given from the inside to allow the softening (as you let go), can you soften the grip of your fascia so that blood can sweep in between the held layers of fascia and muscle and carry away the chemistry that had been trapped there by the freeze response.

We still have so much more to learn about this releasing process. In fact, I accept that we barely begin to comprehend the countless complex and amazing processes that take place throughout the human body as it adapts, copes, and survives. But I'm very familiar with the phenomenon of buried memories escaping to the surface when a practitioner is working with the fascia in myofascial release.

What You Resist Persists

As the body responds to our use of it, layers of cells thicken throughout areas that are repeatedly "loaded"; that is, areas where we bear weight or where force is generated. You might have heard what is now becoming a common adage: "What you resist persists" in the realm of psychology. This can be applied to fascia, too. When fascia in these loaded areas fortifies itself to withstand the effects of the loading, it is this form of resistance that creates a persistence. That is, if holding patterns are left uninterrupted, we can eventually become frozen in our own resistance as, over time, the fascia ossifies and turns to bone.

An example of this can be seen in "hammer toes" (proper name *hallux malleus*), when the toes take on an appearance of constantly gripping. This can be caused as the body repeatedly corrects for the forward tilt in most shoes caused by even the slightest elevated heel. (Yes, men—your shoes, too, will cause this.)

The torsional force forward causes the body to feel like it is going to tip over and the toes grip in response to prevent this. For an example of what hammer toes look like, search for "Hammer toe" on Wikipedia or scan this QR code:

An elevated heel throws off our alignment by transferring our weight from the heels into the toes. In addition, a flip-flop that doesn't have a strap extending far enough back to keep it on our foot, causes the toes to contract automatically to keep the sandal on, which creates an unconscious gripping pattern.

The toes eventually "freeze" in that pattern, and can no longer be straightened unless a surgeon breaks the bones and resets them. Even then, if corrections aren't made to adjust the body mechanics that caused the gripping, the toes can calcify again.

One of the goals of myofascial release is to bring a client's awareness to the areas where holding patterns are strangling nerves and blood vessels. It's like opening your fascial "fishnet" to make the weave wider, so that as you move through life, energy that is coming *at* you can flow *through* you and not get stuck *in* you.

I'll illustrate this by the following two accounts of injuries to my own body. In the first, I did my best to recover quickly, having no idea how to let myself feel and release the fear I felt at the moment of impact. In the second, I knew that trying to suppress my feelings would create resistance and further holding patterns in my body. The two outcomes were very different.

The Time I Got Hit By a Car

When I was twelve, and knew everything, I was allowed to walk from our house into town—a distance of about three miles.

One summer day I had a friend over. We were home alone at my house, and got bored. We decided to walk downtown to buy some candy, so we raided my mom's penny jar.

On the way home from our little jaunt, I thought it would be a great idea, rather than wait for the traffic light, to just dash between the cars stopped for the red light and head for the other side of the road. I motioned for my friend to come with me, but she was smart enough not to follow.

I can only imagine what it was like, for the young fellow and his girlfriend who had just started accelerating from the green light, to see me dart out in front of them. The car had gotten up to only about fifteen miles an hour when I appeared so suddenly that they couldn't avoid hitting me.

The impact was to my right hip. It bounced me in the air, and knocked the wind out of me as I hit the street.

When I could focus again, I was looking up at the sky. The smell of the warm asphalt was strong. A crowd of people had gathered around me, and a gas station worker with hands stained black was telling me to bite his finger. A true hero in action, he thought I might have a seizure, and had heard somewhere that you were supposed to give the victim something to bite on. Even in my daze, I politely declined.

Then I heard an ambulance arrive, and I remember just feeling stupid. *Oh, man—my parents are going to be so mad at me.*

To this day I don't know how they handled getting my friend back home to where she belonged. I'm so sorry about that day, Debbie, wherever you are now. How awful that must have been for you to witness.

I don't remember a lot of pain. I do remember a lot of fear.

Once I arrived in the emergency room, nurses had to cut off my brand-new floral print denim shorts—more upsetting to me, at the time, than how my body felt.

In those days before cell phones, my parents couldn't be immediately contacted. I remember staring at the ceiling on a gurney in a dark hallway, waiting alone for the X-ray tech to come take a picture of my bones.

Afterward, he handed me a cup of flat Coca-Cola. I was scandalized, because this was a forbidden beverage according to my religion, but I was thirsty and no one was there to shame me about it, so I gulped it down.

The X-rays showed a hairline fracture of my pelvis, and I was treated to several days in the hospital. I got letters from the kids in my class and a board game from my teacher, Ms. Kaiser, entitled "Go to the Head of the Class." I remember wondering if this was a secret message that I was her pet. (It wasn't.)

I was released to go home on crutches, and for a couple of weeks I hobbled around on them by putting more weight on my left foot, until I got the doctor's okay to start bearing weight again.

Throughout this event and its aftermath, I wanted to apologize. I was focused on the embarrassment of having made a really obvious mistake, and I didn't want my parents to be mad at me. I didn't want the hospital bill to be expensive, and didn't want the poor kids who had been driving the car to feel bad about themselves.

I have no memory of shaking or crying or taking the opportunity to let my body tell the truth about how that experience felt and how it affected me.

To this day, my left leg still wants to take ultimate responsibility, and when I'm not paying attention it carries more of my weight.

The Time I Injured My Right Foot

In my forties, I had a foot injury. I had been persuaded that a Vespa scooter was a good idea, and I didn't avail myself of any training before hopping on this thing and riding around the corner to an appointment.

Once there, I realized that I'd forgotten something important at home, but I knew I could hop back on my scooter, dash back to my house, retrieve the missing item, and quickly get back for my appointment.

What I didn't count on was the driver backing up in the parking lot I was scooting through. I cleverly avoided being hit by squeezing my brakes, laying the bike down, and sliding across the asphalt on my right side.

Time slowed down in that moment of terror, and it seemed that the slide would never end.

While my helmet protected my head, and my jeans protected my leg, I was wearing sandals. My foot was underneath the scooter and could go nowhere. It just took everything the unyielding asphalt had to offer.

When I finally slid to a stop, I lay there for a moment.

I wanted to hop up and say, "I'm fine!" I tried, and for a moment actually thought I was being convincing.

I saw two women get out of the car and hurry toward me. It seemed weird that they looked so much alike and were speaking with English accents. It's funny the things that imprint themselves on your memory during times of trauma, versus the things you don't remember at all.

Then my vision started to narrow until I could see only a white dot, and I ended up laid out on the grass, staring up at the sky again.

The driver and her sister must have felt terrible. One of them kept saying, "I didn't see you. I didn't see you."

The EMTs arrived, and one of them was extremely good-looking, with black hair (instead of black fingers) and blue eyes, like Superman. They wanted to cut my pants off again! This time I wouldn't let them.

Because I didn't want to incur the ambulance fee, I let an onlooker drive me the short distance to the hospital, where I was treated for lacerations and road rash. The wound over the joint of my right big toe was stitched closed. On the top of my foot there wasn't enough skin left to stitch together, so that was left open to heal, and I was ultimately left with a circular scar there. No X-rays were taken, and it wasn't discovered till later that the right big toe had been broken at the joint, so it just healed while I hobbled on it.

I returned to work later that week. As a single mother needing to make a living, I didn't want the fancy spa resort to know that I was crippled. Luckily, white Crocs were an acceptable part of the uniform, so I cut away the top area of the shoe that would touch the wound, and my pants covered it.

I faked it that way until one of the managers saw the injury. I was sent home, and told not to return without a note from my doctor. The wound on the top of my foot was so deep that it took forever to heal; it was eight weeks before I could get back to work.

This time around, however, I allowed myself to pitch a fit. I would wait until everyone was out of the house and then I'd cry and wail, rolling back and forth on my bed and saying all the things I'd held in.

"It's not fair!"

"I don't like this!"

"It's not my fault!"

"Get me out of here!"

"I want to slap somebody!"

"I'm a good person. Why me?"

"Who do I talk to about this?"

"Somebody needs to fix this!"

I growled and snarled, knowing that, without witnesses, my behavior couldn't possibly go on my permanent record. I wasn't afraid to let my animal nature fully express how it felt about the suddenness and pain and injustice of it all.

Doing this felt exquisite.

I always ended up sleeping pretty soundly after a fit, and can say that I have few residual effects from that accident.

Chapter Five
When Fascia Is Injured

I will discuss two distinct types of possible injury to your fascia. One type can be caused by micro-tears to the fibers (designated by the suffix *-itis*, as in tendonitis), and the other can be caused by derangement of the fibers (indicated by the suffix *-osis*, as in tendonosis).

Each cell in your body contains chemicals of inflammation. When tissues are damaged, the cells rupture and these inflammatory chemicals (called macrophages) release insulin-like growth factor 1 (IGF-1) to help the injured tissue to heal. In other words, inflammation is a good thing. However, an injured area might have a tightening of the fascia from a freeze response, restricting the flow of blood and lymph through the area. This can invite too much inflammation, resulting in adhesions and scarring.

In the acute stage when an area of tissue has just been damaged, the inflammatory process begins. As the inflammation heals the tissues, an overproduction of repair cells can create a derangement (or tangle) of the fascia.

In other words, *–itis* can lead to *–osis*. This causes a reduction in tensile strength and range of motion in the fascia. A weakened area like this, known as a "stress riser," makes a subsequent injury more likely to occur in the area surrounding an initial injury.

Surgery causes a derangement of fascial tissues. If myofascial release is administered as soon as possible after a surgery or tear, it will encourage the repairing fibroblasts to arrange themselves in the same direction as the muscle instead of haphazardly around the wound. This lowers the risk of a stress riser being created.

What a Doctor Will Do

We visit doctors with a complaint of pain and an expectation that they'll make it go away *right now*. Physicians are highly motivated to do that. They have an arsenal of drugs they can prescribe that will reduce the inflammation and the sensation that we're feeling. These are corticosteroids and nonsteroidal anti-inflammatory drugs (NSAIDs such as acetaminophen, ibuprofen, aspirin, etc).

However, aside from dulling the pain, these drugs destroy our collagen-based connective tissue, and this has been known in the medical field and printed in the medical literature for decades.

I want to emphasize that a preponderance of studies have shown that this number one treatment for the inflammatory complaint of osteoarthritis (OA) *actually causes worsening over time*. The growing medical consensus is that this mode of treatment should have been discontinued decades ago.

Rather than turn off the pain signal, we want to increase blood flow to the area by releasing the squeeze of our fascial fishnet with gentle traction, stretching, and compression. This will ease the strangulation of blood supply to the tissue, allowing flow in and out of the area so that the inflammatory process is no longer thwarted.

In addition to stretching and myofascial release, consider another inexpensive, long-term, superior alternative to the debilitating results of NSAIDs, prescription painkillers, and their side effects. Eat a healthy diet. Though the effects may not be as immediate as those of MFR, we can improve our eating habits and consciously choose foods that supply our fascia with what it needs to repair and to remain healthy. I'll go into this further in Chapter Seven.

Think Twice Before You Ice

I was born in San Diego, California. When I was four, we moved to Hudson, Massachusetts, where the climate change was a shock to my system. While living in New England, I always felt as if something were wrong. My young body had absolutely no love of the cold. I didn't like having to put on layers and layers of clothing that were never enough to keep away the chill.

I remember how odd it was to be sweating under my clothes, yet with my face so numb that I was unable to feel my lips. I was baffled when my mouth couldn't form words anymore; it just wouldn't move right. My whole body ached and shivered for what seemed like seven months out of the year.

Since becoming an a-fascia-nado, I now understand why being cold is so painful. It makes our connective tissue lose elasticity and our collagen hardens!

When I was fourteen, my father was hired in the Silicon Valley. We moved back to California, and I've been inviting the sun to warm my formerly frozen fascia ever since.

In Western medicine, the gold standard for treatment of injury has, until recently, been the acronym RICE. It stands for rest, ice, compression, and elevation, as put forth by Dr. Gabe Mirkin in 1978. In March of 2014, on his own website at drmirkin.com/fitness/why-ice-delays-recovery.html, Dr. Mirkin reversed himself, citing the many recent studies that show how ice actually slows the healing process.

Try telling that to the die-hard enthusiasts of RICE. They not only aren't open to hearing it; they become downright emotional about it and are ready to "throw down" with anyone who disagrees. The science speaks for itself, though.

In explaining the reversal of his former recommendation, Dr. Mirkin began by saying, "Coaches have used my 'RICE' guideline for decades, but now it appears that both ice and complete rest may delay healing, instead of helping."

He cited the January 2004 issue of *The American Journal of Sports Medicine*, which provided a summary of twenty-two scientific articles showing many research studies that found almost no evidence that ice and compression helped healing over the use of compression alone. Here's the QR code for that web page:

When connective tissue gets cold, it loses its elasticity and the interstitial fluid that fills all the spaces between the body structures thickens. As Dr. Mirkin pointed out, when you apply ice to reduce swelling, it constricts blood vessels near the injury and thus shuts off the flow of blood that carries the macrophages that release IGF-1 to repair the injured tissue. Your blood vessels won't reopen for many hours after the application of ice. This decrease in blood supply can cause the tissue to die, leading to permanent damage.

Dr. Mirkin recommends that if pain is acute, it is acceptable to apply ice as a temporary, short-term measure, but he adds that, if more than six hours have passed after an injury, there is no reason to apply ice.

Chapter Six
Instinct Is Forever

The body comes equipped with factory-installed voluntary and involuntary responses. When we're babies, we involuntarily poop and pee. As we mature, that function comes more and more under our voluntary control—sometimes to the point where the body just won't allow us to poop anywhere but at home!

But we never mature so much that we no longer need to poop and pee; if you try to hold it in too long, your body will have its release without your permission.

The physical reaction to fearful stimuli is involuntary, although, to a considerable extent, we learn to bring it under voluntary control. When we hear a sudden loud noise, we startle in reaction. Our animal instinct is then to brace against perceived danger and clamp down in the freeze response.

If we have no awareness that this is a function of our fascia, we're simply at the mercy of it. But having an understanding of how the connective tissue works gives us the power, through awareness, to control our reactions.

We will never mature to the point that we don't have this animal-instinct reaction. For our survival, we need to jump, move, and react when we're frightened. The muscles that react first are the two psoas muscles—one on each side of the spine, running down to the groin—that lift the legs for fight or flight. In plural, the psoas major and psoas minor muscles are the *psoai* (pronounced "so-eye").

The psoai are some of the largest and thickest muscles in the body; on average, each psoas is sixteen inches long. They attach to all five lumbar vertebrae as well as to the intervertebral discs of the low back, and extend forward over the pelvis, finally attaching at the big bone (femur) of the upper leg or groin area. This makes twenty-two attachments: twenty points on the spine plus one on each thigh.

Cavewoman, Adrenaline, and You

Cavewoman (Caveman, too) used to be able to have an honest reaction to adrenaline. She would round a corner, unexpectedly encounter a threatening wild animal, and react. Inside her body the little adrenal glands sitting on top of her kidneys would release a shot of adrenaline straight to her psoas muscles.

Cavewoman would then be ready to kick, scratch, bite, and run, and she would do it. In the process, her muscular use would interrupt the fascial squeeze and help move the acid bath off the surface of the muscles, to metabolize away all of that chemistry.

The next time she emptied her bladder, her urine would contain the chemicals produced by her fear response and muscular use: adrenaline, uric acid, and lactic acid.

Modern woman, when she's driving and someone suddenly pulls out in front of her, still gets the same amount of adrenaline flushed into her system as Cavewoman did. However, the only reactive movement she allows herself is to quickly shift her foot from the accelerator to the brake.

She has within her a strong need to inhibit any wild response to the adrenaline. If she were to kick and flail, she'd further endanger herself and others. She's essentially telling her body *Not now*, in the freeze response. The mechanism that then kicks in to inhibit her movement is the fascial web, which squeezes in like a sea anemone, trapping the adrenaline between the psoas and other muscles and their surrounding sleeves of fascia.

What happens next is important. Modern woman still has a half hour of driving before she arrives home. By the time she gets there, if she hasn't forgotten the incident she processes it intellectually: "Some jerk cut me off and nearly killed us all." And then she dismisses it. But she doesn't realize that her body is still holding its response to that moment of fear.

She's been taught to act like a grownup, so she suppresses the urge to let her body tell the truth and react to the adrenaline now trapped by fascia against the surface of her psoas muscles. If her fear-induced physical freeze response goes uninterrupted, each psoas is left to marinate in that encapsulated cocktail of chemistry.

As I've explained, in that frozen state, blood can't flow between the layers and carry away fear's chemical byproducts, which start to crystallize and get gummy, acting like glue and causing restriction as the layer of fascia adheres to the layer of muscle.

You might have heard the term *adhesions* used by those in the field of rehabilitation and massage. Those are the restrictions in fascia that have accumulated from a lifetime of telling your body *Not now*. What that feels like to an MFR practitioner working with your body is something hard and tight and maybe even crunchy. What that feels like to you is soreness, pain, and a restricted range of motion.

A Severe Lack of Temper Tantrums

Many of us are going about our life without any interruption of the fight-or-flight response in our body. Diagnoses of restless leg syndrome and post-traumatic stress disorder are being used to describe what many are experiencing as an inability to sleep, hold still, or let go of trauma.

At some point, the freeze response must be interrupted so the parasympathetic nervous system can kick in for the rest-and-restore response. Awareness of this truth can give you the power to choose, the option to exert conscious intention to interrupt the holding patterns through movement, stretching, and myofascial release . . . or a good temper tantrum.

You might not realize the value of a temper tantrum. That's not to say that you should have one in front of everybody. But if you knew that you could go to your bedroom, close the door, lie on the bed, and begin gently kicking your heels against the mattress and pounding your fists just to get it started, you might work your way into a full-on physical release of that stored energy, having decided that *Okay . . . now* it's time to let go and clean out all that stored acidity.

The best temper tantrum happens soon after a fright, and is like that of a two-year-old. It involves kicking, rolling around, punching the mattress, screaming into a pillow, and just allowing caveman or cavewoman to tell the truth about how his or her body and emotions felt at the time of the incident. This can provide what's needed to empty out and metabolize away all that encapsulated chemistry.

This could be a daily cleansing habit. It doesn't matter whether you know any of the reasons why you're having this physical discharge of energy. You don't have to worry that you're going crazy or that you'll get so worked up you won't be able to regain your sanity.

In fact, for those who think that this just reinforces a negative pattern, I challenge you to try to sustain a physical release. It has a short shelf life, coming and going like a summer squall. And when it's spent, you're empty. This is so much better than waiting till you have an excuse to "go off" when you stub your toe, drop something and break it, or overreact when someone says something offensive.

The stored energy needs to come out somehow. Some use running, gardening, journaling, or bungee jumping as their pressure release valve. Why not have conscious awareness of this need in your body, let go of ideas about dignity and appropriateness, and have yourself a safe, great, private, grand ol' snit fit? You could call it your snit-fitness program.

Cats and Dogs Know Myofascial Release

Find a pet and press your thumb into its haunch. Your dog or cat couldn't care less. But I challenge you to do that to the hip muscle of an average human being, because you can count on a big reaction.

Cats and dogs know how to do a long myofascial stretch when they get up from a nap. We used to do that when we were little. Remember a Saturday morning when you had nowhere you had to be? Perhaps you slept in and allowed yourself to indulge in that slow awakening, followed by a long stretch that culminates in a squeal and a shiver?

At some point a schedule was imposed, deadlines were established, and you had to wake up to an alarm clock. As you progressed toward adulthood, you probably thought that, the more you skipped over the slow awakening and the stretch, the more responsible you were learning to be.

If we only remembered to do that kind of stretching every day as animals do, three times a day, we could unlock a "physical reset" instinct that clears space and draws light further into our constricted fascial tubules.

Forming the Mask

Because our ability to live in community is imperative to our survival, we learn to adapt, fit in, get along, and negotiate to get our needs met and thrive. This requires frequent adjustments to many different situations.

One of the ways we adapt is by forming masks. We learn to make subtle adaptations to our face to hide any expression that would interfere with us getting our needs met.

These patterns become deeply ingrained. An automatic greeting of, "Hey, how are you?" is met by the automatic response, "Fine," accompanied by an adjustment of the face that's meant to match.

You'd be surprised to know how much tension you carry in your face. It's rare that you allow your features to return to neutral. Try this experiment.

First, wash your hands. Then, using the thumb of your right hand, place it in your mouth and press outward on your left cheek until you begin to feel resistance at the corner of your left nostril. Sustain that for a moment.

You can feel how much holding you had there, and how good it feels to get a little stretch in that area. You don't have to understand why; you just know it feels good.

It's important to your overall health that you bring your awareness to holding patterns like this and grant your body permission to interrupt them. The tissues of not only your face, but your whole body, are starving for this.

My Zero-Gravity Fall

We bought some really cool lawn chairs that were promoted as "zero gravity." I enjoyed sitting in them—especially at night, because I could simply lean back and the chair would recline until my body was nearly supine. Then I could watch the sky for shooting stars.

On one such occasion, I thought that, instead of leaving my legs out straight, I would cross them, Indian-style. I didn't know that the chair wouldn't support this activity. Boom! Backward it fell, and my head and back landed hard on the ground.

I didn't see that coming. It scared me and knocked the wind out of me. I was stunned and unsure how to react.

Joe, my hero and partner in business and life, was with me, and he reminded me about what I teach. He said, "Don't try to get up right away. Hang out there for a minute and pitch a fit."

This was great advice! I allowed myself to shout, "That scared me! I didn't like that! I hurt myself! I'm a good person—it isn't fair!" And I flailed my arms and kicked my feet, allowing that shock to move through me.

I'm happy to report that I suffered no lasting ill effects from that event, and I can even say that I'm grateful to have these occasional opportunities to practice what I preach.

Chapter Seven
MFR Is More Than Just Physical

At this point, you might be giving thought to the idea of receiving some myofascial work. I applaud that possibility, because I encourage everyone to begin this inward exploration.

Even though you might have previously considered *feeling* as *weakness*, it is actually *strength and empowerment*. Think of the energy to be regained from releasing all of that fascial holding it's taken to keep yourself "appropriate."

Getting the Most from Treatment

I want to describe what MFR treatments can entail, so that you can get the most from them.

During a session of myofascial release, the practitioner provides sustained traction or compression on the client's skin, moving in the direction of ease until he or she feels a stopping point. Here, the therapist maintains an intention for release, waiting patiently for the collagen and elastin components of the fascia to eventually melt, stretch, and elongate.

The weave of the fascia begins to widen. When the traction is held long enough, this provides an opportunity for an unconscious holding pattern to come into the client's awareness. As the therapist maintains the invitation to let go, the person on the table begins to notice the resistance coming from within. Some experience the feeling of trying to let go and finding that their body doesn't remember how.

It helps to direct your mind with the conscious thought, *Nothing bad will happen if I let go*. As you calm the feeling of panic, this can wake up the parasympathetic response. The fascia can let go of its "protect and defend" mode and reset to "safe and soft."

As the holding pattern eases and the fascia lengthens, blood begins to seep between the layers of fascia and muscle, and the stuck places that were glued to each other begin to open, expand, and let go, allowing the blood to sweep away those old, acidic byproducts of fear.

As that fear cocktail is flushed into your bloodstream, you experience the feelings triggered by that released chemistry: fear, grief, anger, panic, sadness, anxiety, and so forth.

Luckily, you don't have to assign a reason to these feelings; you just need to let your body feel and express them so it can eliminate all of the stored fear chemistry that has been taking up space and energy in your body and causing your internal organs to compress and stick together.

When your body starts to let go and you feel a negative emotion, your intellect may want to stop the feeling from being expressed. Have you ever been dreaming that you need to pee, and in your dream you finally find a toilet, sit down on it, and start to let go? A strong pattern wakes you up to remind you that it's not okay to pee in bed.

In a similar way, as your intellect begins to step back and let your body lead the way, and as you then start to let go of your internal clenching, your interfering mind can reawaken and try to regain control.

Your intellect may tell you that only crazy people act this way, or that you're out of control and need to rein it in, or that, if you start down that road, you may not be able to stop, or that people are watching or this is dangerous for your very survival and ability to fit in and be protected by your village.

If this happens, you have an opportunity to thank your intellect for sharing and enlist its cooperation, letting it know that this is not an intellectual pursuit but a feeling one. Fascial release is not within the domain of the intellect. Tell your mind that, to deal with the panic response, rather than bracing, it will better serve you to develop a new pattern of softening.

Feeding Your Fascia

Now that we're learning how crucially important and physically omnipresent fascia is, maybe it's time to take into consideration the health of our connective tissue right along with the well-being of the rest of our body.

Fascia is made of collagen and elastin. The nutrients that nourish this connective tissue include:

- Omega-3 in the form of pure grade fish oil.
- Collagen from leafy green vegetables and red fruits. Vitamins C, B and E and phytoestrogens that promote collagen production.
- Calcium found in almond and coconut milk.
- Chondroitin, found in animal tissue along with Glucosamine, found in animal marrow. A supplement would be the more likely source for this.
- Methylsulfonylmethane (MSM), found in vegetables that are rich in the colors green, red, orange and yellow.

It makes good sense, then, to include every one of these foods and supplemental nutrients in our diet. As your body interacts with the nutrition it receives, the thought patterns you carry, and all the variables in your gravitational environment, all of these factors contribute to the patterns that form in your body.

How Physical Holding Gets Developed

Imagine that you're standing in front of your car, looking at the tires, and you notice that they're not mounted straight. The right one is pointing to the right, and the left one is pointing to the left.

Would you continue to drive your car that way? If you did, you could expect many things to wear out, due to the forces exerted upon the misaligned structures.

Yet many people walk with their feet turned outward. Their knees follow this outward turn as well, no longer facing forward in the direction they intend to walk. So, since a knee can bend in only one direction, these people have to use a subtle inward twist of the upper leg and push off the ground against the joint of the big toe in order to propel themselves in a forward direction. If their weight shifted in the direction their toes are pointing, with each step they would be wasting a lot of energy moving side to side rather than forward.

This movement pattern creates compensatory reactions in the skeleton and soft tissues from the feet to the neck. The soft tissues begin to morph and adapt to support how the body is being used. If such a person now straightens his feet, it flushes out a pattern of internal rotation of the upper leg, with tight, thickened fascia that cause his knees to twist inward toward each other. The classes I teach start with correct foot alignment. Many beginning students remark, "This feels pigeon-toed!"

Further, every time we cast our eyes downward when we're walking, our head shifts out over our toes. It's like hanging a bowling ball over the toes and asking the body to compensate for that forward pull.

Then, with every step we stimulate unwanted bone growth in the forward part of each foot—instead of striking the ground with the large bone of the heel, which is the place designed to take the weight and vibrate the entire skeleton.

Heel strikes stimulate bone growth (osteogenesis) throughout the skeletal structure, as each step vibrates the whole body and not just the tiny bones of our toes.

Bone grows where it is repeatedly loaded with force. Since gravity is always exerting force downward, if our bones are not lined up to resist it, our soft tissues are recruited to keep us from falling forward. A holding pattern of *Uh-oh, we're going to fall forward* becomes ingrained in our soft tissues.

Other holding patterns develop in response to our beliefs. If, as children, we were admonished that it is rude to speak loudly, we probably developed a holding pattern in our throat to quiet our voice. We certainly have been told not to steal other kids toys or slap people, so we have an appropriate holding pattern in our arms.

Some girls are reminded to sit with their knees together and to not wiggle so much when they walk. Boys learn to "suck it up" when they get hurt and to not react with any "girly" tears. A practical knowledge of fascia gives you the awareness to interrupt these patterns regularly, in order to avoid becoming an acidic storage tank of unreleased movement and emotion.

Human Patterns

I love puzzles because, for me, they're just like getting a box of snarled fascia and having the opportunity to smooth it all out till it fits together and presents a cohesive picture.

In putting together a puzzle, I follow the patterns that help me flesh out the bigger picture, just as I do in my work.

No matter how disorganized we might think ourselves to be, we follow patterns all day, every day. Think for just a moment about the ways in which you follow a pattern. You'll find a pattern in the way you get up and get dressed and fix your hair and get ready for work. You'll also find a pattern in the way you go to bed. There are patterns in the way you argue . . . in the way you walk and talk and learn and eat. Your body has nerve patterns and fibrous patterns and emotional patterns and circulatory patterns. The very way you breathe follows a pattern.

We can sometimes influence these patterns. But, when they're not in our conscious awareness, there's nothing we can do about them. The moment you bring your attention to a pattern, you can influence it. Since my focus is on fascia, I want to emphasize all of the good things that happen when we interrupt our holding patterns.

During treatment, we have no need to grip harder to suppress our feelings, no need to interpret feeling our emotions as being dangerous, out of control or insane. For once, we can let go . . . the body is emptying itself of that stagnant old chemistry.

Clients will often say, "This is the stuff I've been trying my whole life *not* to feel. Why would you ask me to do this?"

I remind them that, as the body releases that toxicity, they're not saying hello to a whole new set of feelings. They're saying goodbye to that old, stagnant chemistry that's being flushed out of the tissues and into the renal system for elimination.

Hydration is important to facilitate the elimination of toxins, so increasing your water intake before a session is something you'll want to remind yourself to do. The water that surrounds the fascia can be characterized as "bulk" water (polluted by inflammatory cells and free radicals), and you want the clean supply of water that will be squeezed from your blood plasma, instantly forming *bound water* zones during treatment.

Bound water is any amount of water in the body tissues that is bound to macromolecules or organelles. It forms a thin, coherent layer around tissues. As the water bonds chemically with other molecules to form this layer, the energy of the water molecule is reduced and can't support microbial growth, participate in chemical reactions, or cause physical changes.

Most textbooks ignore the presence of water in your organs, muscles, and tissues. Yet, seeing living fascia gives you a visual understanding of the importance of water in your fascia and makes it obvious that studying fascia on cadavers did *not* give us a complete picture or allow us to see fascia's fiber-optic nature when it's plumped and full of fluid.

As Dr. Pollack explains, the water in our cells and blood is not like water in a glass. A fourth phase of water exists, not H^2O but H^3O^2, and this can be called living water. It's more viscous, dense, and alkaline than regular water. It has a negative charge, and can hold and deliver energy, much like a battery.

When cellular water interacts with the charged surfaces of our tissues, the molecules become structured in arrays of strata and the water becomes liquid-crystalline with an H^3O^2 molecular structure.

If you'd like to gain a deeper understanding of this, I recommend that you read *The Fourth Phase of Water: Beyond Solid, Liquid, and Vapor* by the scientist Gerald H. Pollack.

You might also search on YouTube for "The Fourth Phase of Water" or scan this QR code:

Drinking more water *after* a session will just happen. Obey your thirst. Fascia is two-thirds water, so slake the needs of those tissues that have for so long been dry and compressed and unable to absorb.

With the expansion of your connective tissue, many little interstitial spaces have opened and are ready to be filled with moisture. This accounts for the copious urinating that sometimes occurs after a session as your body releases the old chemistry, and is the reason why you may want to reconsider drinking alcohol or caffeine after a treatment. As your fascial system drinks in the fluid that you provide it, these substances hit you much harder than they usually would.

It's important to note that fear is not the only thing that we store or tell our body *Not now* about. You might have stored silliness, laughter, and joy. That happened to me most often in church, in school, and riding in the car.

You might have received, as my siblings and I did, admonitions to "Be quiet," "Sit down," and "Hold still" when you were being loudly happy. So you might find yourself erupting in paroxysms of laughter while receiving myofascial release, as I sometimes do.

No matter what happens in a session, let me reassure you that while you're receiving treatment you cannot screw it up. You can't get it wrong. This is an easy "A." There are no expectations about your "performance" on the table. There's only you, letting go in places where you're ready and holding on where you're not ready. And everything that happens is leading you away from physical deterioration and toward healing.

Here's the kicker. As your fascia begins to open and let go, the parasympathetic nervous system is turned on. This triggers a release of endorphins, oxytocin, and dopamine—the chemistry of love.

As I leave the treatment room, often the appearance of the person on the table is like that of a wide-open, peacefully sleeping, post-tantrum two-year-old. I think any painter would love to capture that portrait of deep repose.

Intellectual Processing vs. Feeling

In 1979 Gerald Jampolsky, MD, wrote a well-received and widely distributed book called *Love Is Letting Go of Fear*. I have benefitted from this book, and have recommended it to many. Dr. Jampolsky's premise isn't just a concept or a clever way of presenting an idea . . . it's biology, baby!

The effects of letting go are chemically quantifiable and measureable. When you understand your fascia, and care for it properly, stretching and melting it can be *way* more effective than any antidepressant. Whereas trying not to feel . . . is like trying not to be human.

Between 1993 and 1995, I undertook a series of seminars in a program called Lifespring. Finding out, through those seminars, that I was the creator of my own experience was so empowering that my life took a dramatic turn.

I immersed myself in this teaching, and participated in many other workshops as a student and then as a facilitator. To this day, not one moment in my life goes by that I don't call upon what I learned there. I am so grateful. This book would not have been written if I hadn't learned the principles they taught me.

And . . . my butt hurt. Most of my hours of participation were spent sitting in a chair.

The transformation occurred in my mind, spirit, and emotions. But an important piece was still missing. I had no idea at the time, but there would be further transformation to experience. My body still had a story to tell. Just as I had learned in Lifespring, I would find what I was looking for inside me—and not just in a manner of speaking, but literally.

You Can't Heal What You Don't Feel

Talking through an issue is an intellectual pursuit that can *feel* satisfying but that doesn't allow your *body* to tell the truth about how *it* feels.

I often see clients who have received extensive talk therapy. Their belief is that, because they have been able to intellectually process a traumatic experience, they're "over it."

Yet I find that their fascia is still clenched in resistance to letting the animal response hidden on the inside be seen on the outside. Being so long accustomed to exerting control, they don't realize how much energy they're expending in order to maintain the appearance of being "fine."

As time goes by, those tissues deprived of circulation begin to fatigue and cry out. Aches and pains increase, and ease of movement is not what it once was. The clients going through all this don't even realize that the pain in their body today is connected to traumas that might have happened years ago.

If you apply this understanding to the phenomenon of post-traumatic stress disorder (PTSD), you realize that prescription medications to numb the symptoms don't allow a person's body to unwind the physical holding that froze inside them during a trauma or multiple traumas.

The body needs the opportunity to tell its truth . . . to release the fear, rage, horror, and agony in the safe container of the treatment room. A person might have so much animal reaction stored and unreleased inside them that they fear that, if they unleashed it, someone would get hurt.

This is why I always have a large pillow and spare bolsters on hand in my treatment room.

If someone needs to kick, punch, bite, scream, or strangle something, these substitutes can provide exactly the physical release the client needs. I have seen this take place, and it's a profound moment when clients realize that they "went there" and yet nobody got hurt.

In fact, they have divested themselves of a physical straitjacket that was squeezing the very life out of them. Their family is spared the "fallout" (as pent-up expression leaks out when they experience challenges in everyday life) and their fascia can allow them to move past the moments of trauma and flush out the fear chemistry that's been trapped against the surface of the muscles.

In addition, we "evolved" and "civilized" humans all hold in our body a lifetime of repressed physical impulses. Think of all the people you didn't kick, punch, slap, bite, or scream at when the animal in you wanted to. You avoided going to prison, because you exercised restraint. But the prison is inside you—it's being built within the fascial web of your body.

Would Knowing Why Make the Pain Stop?

Let's imagine you're on my treatment table. The story of how each layer of holding came into your body is inaccessible to both of us. A memory may come up as you let go and an area of old chemistry is set free into the bloodstream, but that's only a small piece of the puzzle.

The surrounding areas, when they responded to the pain with the protective biological reaction of tightening, created a maze of holding patterns extending to other areas of your body. Unbeknownst to you, there has been a whole network of reactive protection going on for years.

A natural left-brain impulse to be logical and linear and rational kicks in, and you find yourself wanting to figure out the cause and effect. Let go of that idea.

Your mind can't possibly comprehend the chain of internal reactions that took place in the thousands of hours that have passed since the original injury. You cannot account for the micro-movements and unconscious accommodations that occurred in the seconds, minutes, hours, days, weeks, years, and decades since the frightening experience happened. So don't even try.

"Do you think this pain could be a result of that skiing accident?"

When I hear a question like that, or hear, "Maybe it got this way because of the repetitive movements I do at my job," or "This is probably because I don't exercise," I ask you this; if you understood *why*, would it make the pain go away?

Without an understanding of fascia, it's easy to see how you wouldn't associate an *emotional trauma* from the past with a *physical pain* in the present, or recognize that your loss of a parent or beloved teacher when you were a child could have precipitated your chest pain as an adult. But even if you never make this connection, it matters less than that the trauma find its physical release.

The mind can't fix it. The answer is in the realm of your *physical* intelligence. The body is brilliant in knowing where it needs to let go, if you let it lead. It has the ability to unwind all the painful patterns, if you can ask your intellect to hold back from trying to comprehend it all.

Pain vs. Sensation

When you're on the path of myofascial release and making your way out of feeling numb, you might interpret everything you're now starting to feel as pain.

But, if you categorize all sensation under the broad heading of pain, you might mistakenly conclude that it must be bad and that we should stop. Ordinarily, when you say "Ouch!" your expectation is that whatever is happening should cease.

I have experienced in myself, and seen in clients, an *anticipation* reaction. While receiving MFR I've sometimes been convinced that where or how I was being touched was really about to hurt me, and I started to say "ouch"—only to giggle and admit out loud that it didn't hurt as I thought it was going to.

In life, we have all been hurt. A lot. As the human potential innovator Werner Erhard has said, "If you want to be comfortable, life is not the place to be."

In my work, I observe that we are more accustomed to being braced and prepared for our next encounter with pain than we are to being open and at ease. But we can change that.

On the treatment table, you need to take on a different mindset because you're not being injured. This is where I encourage clients to tune in to exactly what sensation it is that they're feeling.

Using words to describe it that involve location, size, and quality helps give greater body awareness and brings people closer to the ability to calm the panic when they feel sensation.

I will ask, "Where do you feel it?" If they say, "My back," I ask, "Upper, middle, lower?" Once they identify where, I'll ask, "What size is it? Like a book? A loaf of bread? A pencil?" Once they know the size, I'll ask, "Is it sharp? Dull? Constant? Intermittent?" and they always know, once they've been asked.

This information had not been available to them before because they had never brought such specific awareness to it. The questioning technique begins to give them more empowerment in their efforts to let go of their own fascial restrictions. Just by bringing this focused awareness to what it is that they're feeling, they're able to reduce its scope and change its quality.

So, in the interest of allowing the body to express what it needs to express without pushing people beyond where they're ready to go, I find that it helps to agree ahead of time that the word "Halt!" will be honored. By speaking this word, the client can let me know that he or she really wants to me to stop the movement and ease the pressure being applied.

Otherwise, any words can be uttered in the interest of allowing the body to empty out. For instance, *I hate you—ow, ow, ow, ow!* Or *It's not fair!* Can be exactly what needs to be expressed in the process of letting go of long-term holding patterns.

This is because, in a lifetime of being told to *shush, suck it up, quit your whining, big boys don't cry* and *nobody wants to hear that*, a great deal of expression has been withheld, and it takes a lot of energy to hang on to that and store it. The treatment room is the place to let it all fly, knowing that you won't be judged for doing so.

Chapter Eight
Unwinding

I'll always remember a workshop experience I had when I was learning myofascial release. In the John Barnes training, after you practice a freshly learned technique on someone, they immediately practice on you. I had begun to take chances when it was my turn to receive, and I was starting to take John Barnes at his word when he said to *let go*.

I was in a training room where others seemed to be moving and making noise during their turn on the table, and I felt ready to see where my body would take me. Choosing a practice partner, I went first as practitioner. Then it was my turn.

I was lying face up, and the other therapist was at my feet, holding my heels with gentle traction.

John Barnes had explained to us about the *fascial voice*—an area of the body that has been signaling with a sensation that's been going on in the background of our attention but mostly drowned out by external stimuli or dismissed by our telling it *Not now*.

I tuned in to where my body was "talking" the most. I could feel a low-grade ache in my left hip, and was surprised that I had been ignoring a sensation that felt fairly obvious once I tuned out everything else. The fascial voice was like a kid yanking on my skirt and saying "Mom. Mom. Mom. Mom. Mom."

Instead of holding still, I let my left leg move of its own accord. With my eyes closed, I let it stretch out straight and then extend out to the side. Both of my arms began to reach up over my head.

I thought, *I'd be mortified if I ever did this while I was receiving a traditional massage*. But I went with it, and as I began to take up space by expanding my movements, the instructor brought more students to assist.

Soon there was a person for each of my limbs, one for my head, and one at my waist. That's right: six people around that table—just for me!

I wrestled with my self-conscious inner voice that was telling me I was taking up too much time, space, attention, and resources. I politely invited my inner critic to *shush*.

Getting Down

Before I knew what was happening, my freedom of movement had brought me way over to one side of the table, and soon I was being gently assisted to the ground!

I didn't have to brace or stop or apologize or start over. They just went with it and followed my body. I allowed myself to follow it, too. That is to say, I didn't let my internal censor/ monitor/editor interrupt or stop me and require me to "act right."

It really helped to have my eyes closed so I didn't get sensory input. If I had seen any of the expressions on the faces of those helping me, it might have inhibited my internal process. However, I remember opening my eyes at one point and being surprised to see the underside of the massage table with all its riggings and wires.

For some reason, this view from the floor filled me with the giddiest sense of euphoria. I was so far outside the box that I was under it! I hadn't even known this was an option. At that moment, what came out of my mouth in a whisper was, "I had no idea," and it felt good for me to repeat these words over and over again. The statement felt like part of the unwinding.

I felt a loosening of all of the physical and mental limits and controls put on me from a young age by my parents and grandparents and their church and my school and teachers and education, and by *me* when I got old enough to take over imposing the constraints on my own. This felt like a return to innocence, a return to my authentic self.

As I kept uttering that one phrase, "I had no idea," the instructor got right down there with me and whispered in my ear, "But what if you *did*?" Just writing these words makes me weep. I wouldn't be writing this, and wouldn't be able to share this beautiful information about *you*, if I hadn't learned that, back then, about *me*.

Throughout my life, the freeze response that had taken place in moments of trauma had stopped my body from having a physical reaction to the fight-or-flight signal firing in my gut. Allowing your body to have the physical expression of fight or flight in a safe environment can unlock long-term patterns of holding. Pounding your heels, cycling your legs, flailing your arms, punching a pillow, and screaming and cursing is an authentic expression of fear that can empty out what your body has stored.

And it's fascinating, because it doesn't happen out of any conscious choice. No one can tell you that you need to scream or repeat phrases like, *I wanna go home.* It just happens when you take the brakes off.

Huge resistance to letting go like this is common. I'll tell you more about this in the next chapter.

When It Wants to Happen, Let It

Fascial unwinding is a spontaneous movement response that sometimes occurs while a client is receiving myofascial release. It can be one of the most beneficial aspects of MFR.

On the treatment table, we can never know when unwinding is going to happen. It often takes place when you're able to let go of worrying about how you look or what noises you're making or why your body is choosing to move in the way that it is.

It can be glorious to open your eyes after a treatment session and find yourself upside down and backwards following movement that started with a stretch and then opened into an expansion that felt so good, so right.

Unwinding can feel like crawling out of a cocoon, like coming back to life. You'd be amazed how good it feels to shake and squeak and twist and yawn and shiver and maybe scream and cry and laugh and spread your toes and push with all your might against the therapist's hands.

That range of physical release comes from the person on the table, not from the practitioner. And bear in mind that the client isn't "right" if they achieve this, or "wrong" if they don't. When it comes to unwinding, there's no need to assign credit or blame; it's all good.

Chapter Nine
"I'm Not Like That."

Carved into the forecourt of Apollo's temple at Delphi is the maxim "Know thyself." In the grand unfolding of your life, there is much self-knowledge to be gained, and much power in the wisdom that you acquire.

We have all learned too well to follow the admonitions to sit down, be quiet, and hold still. So we put up "drywall" in our thinking: those hard, steadfast, unexamined rules about what "normal" is and the proper way to act.

Can you think of any areas that *you* have cordoned off? Areas represented by restrictive phrases like the following have, through the ages, given rise to a lot of physical unease:

"Nice girls don't."

"We don't talk about that."

"Suck it up."

"A sane person would never behave that way."

We all believe falsehoods about life and about ourselves that are strong and resistant to change. I find rigid thinking to be an especially common trait among clients who have a great deal of myofascial pain and holding in their body.

I want them to know that the rules are different in the treatment room. After I describe to them the kinds of things that can occur when the intellect gets out of the way and the body has permission to tell the truth of how it feels about its lifetime of experience, we play a game to fill in the blanks.

Filling in the Blanks

During treatment, the closing of the door to the outside world allows you to expand your parameters to fully occupy the space. As you lie there with your eyes closed, tuning in to the fascial voice, you're free to just *be*, and feel, without apology—without worrying about being polite or appropriate or politically correct.

I assure clients that nothing expressed through word, sound, or movement will be judged or taken personally. This is their opportunity to look to their own needs, for once, and to allow their awareness to permeate their body. I encourage any instinct to move, because such movement can be five times more beneficial than any single thing I can do with traction or compression.

"I'm not like that," they'll say. I kind of know that already; that's why they're here.

Each client's body has a lifetime of appropriateness stored up. Because we have only ourselves for comparison, we tend to think that everyone else shares certain common beliefs (as evidenced by phrases like *You don't just . . . Nobody likes it when . . . It isn't easy to . . .* as if these are accepted truths that everybody knows).

So, to help clients uncover hidden beliefs and start to break through some of the drywall in their thinking, I've learned to ask for their participation with some fill-in-the-blank statements. Here are examples of the kinds of statements I'll initiate and let people complete, to help them flush out the thought patterns behind their physical holding:

"A person who makes a lot of noise is . . . "

"Somebody who flails about is . . ."

"A person who cries is . . . "

"Someone who's angry is . . . "

"Anyone who curses is . . . "

"I'm afraid if I let go . . . "

"If I lose control, I'm afraid I might . . ."

"The worst thing that could happen if I let go is . . ."

"It's better to be quiet because . . ."

"I don't feel anything because . . ."

There are no right or wrong answers, of course. Most people have never thought about these "issues in their tissues," and aren't aware of the judgments and beliefs they hold in their mind that have caused the tightening in their body.

I'm guessing that, in reading those, you might have been filling in some of the blanks for yourself. Explorations like these can lead to some great personal realizations.

"Know thyself." Because, the more you do, the more conscious can be the choices that you make.

Prices and Payoffs

Not everyone responds positively to myofascial release. Holding patterns are not the only thing that's unconscious, as there can be a number of unconscious psychological reasons why you experience pain.

In your process of discovery, you might find that certain perks have come with your having received a diagnosis. These payoffs are pretty universal, so why not just "out" some of them right now?

- People feel sympathy for you.
- It makes you unique and special.
- It can give you a great reason to rest or quit your job.
- It can make you feel important.
- You might be identifying with a parent or role model.
- It might bring you attention or hold someone close to you.
- It might be a legitimate pathway to prescription drugs.
- You might be avoiding meeting your true potential.
- It might help you avoid commitment.
- It might help you avoid growing up.
- It can provide you with security, especially if you are legally declared permanently disabled.

- It might be a way to punish someone whom you feel has hurt you.
- It might be what gives you a sense of identity.
- It might be a way of making yourself "right."

You might be able to add some others that came to mind as you were reading this.

When faced with the prospect of letting go and finding the pathway out of all that holding and pain, you might begin to feel a great sense of loss for something that has become so familiar and provided you with one or several of the listed payoffs.

Your support system can be thrown for a loop, too. Partners and caregivers might have become identified with their role, and might feel threatened by the changes they experience as their loved one begins to improve and needs them less or becomes less easy to control.

Switching Your Genes On or Off

Your genes do not turn themselves on and off. Movement, nutrition, emotions, environment, and thoughts create the chemical reactions that switch genes on or off. These factors, called *epigenetics*, have been known for decades.

Thanks to the videos, teaching, and published work of the microbiologist Bruce Lipton, PhD, this understanding started to take shape in the 1990s after the inception of an international scientific research project.

Once this study, called the Human Genome Project, was under way, scientists began to realize that there are fewer human genes than they had thought.

In order to support the theory that genes *control* biology, there would have to be at least one hundred twenty thousand genes in the makeup of a human. In fact, there are thought to be only twenty thousand to twenty-five thousand, and as gene-finding methods are improved it may be found that there are even fewer.

We can no longer attribute our health just to genetic predisposition. Unfortunately, it still takes ten to fifteen years for scientific findings to make it into textbooks so that the new information can be sent out in all directions via the Internet and can become public knowledge.

The bottom line: Genes determine your height, blood type, handedness (left or right), and the color of your hair, eyes, and skin, but they don't control your biology. And even if you do have a genetic marker for a particular disease, it won't necessarily manifest in your body unless there happens to be a chemical environment to switch it on.

You Can Stop Blaming Genetics

Have you ever said, "It runs in our family"? Somewhere along the way, you might have picked up this pattern of thought, and it could now be draining away some of your personal power.

The "runs-in-our-family" statement can cause you to stop right where you are. It can keep you from inquiring any further and can make you feel like a victim. It's also unlikely to be based in fact. If you have a diagnosis that has caused you to think of an illness as inevitable and beyond your control, it's worth finding out if there really is a genetic marker for it.

In his book *The Biology of Belief: Unleashing the Power of Consciousness, Matter, and Miracles*, Dr. Bruce Lipton opened our minds to the idea that our beliefs influence our genes and DNA.

To date, only four genetic diseases are known to affect the fascia: Marfan syndrome, Ehlers-Danlos syndrome, Epidermolysis bullosa (EB), and the inherited disease Alport syndrome. Unless you've been tested for and then diagnosed as having one of these four, there's no reason to believe that your fascia is resistant to healing.

You have the power to effect change in your tissues.

The belief, "I have bunions. My mother had bunions, and my grandmother had them; therefore bunions are hereditary," is inaccurate. Increased bone density in the joint of your big toe occurs due to increased weight bearing in that area of the foot.

There is no genetic marker for bunions, which are no more determined by your genes than your dialect is. The way you pronounce "quarter" or "aluminum" is not a result of your genes. We survive on instinct, and we have a strong human instinct to imitate. The family you grew up with and the region you grew up in provided the model you learned to copy.

Watch a small boy walking next to his dad and you may smile as you notice him imitating his father's gait. A client once told me that his father's polio had caused a limp. As a child, he began to imitate his admired dad's walk, and he distinctly remembers his father scolding him, saying, "Stop walking like me and imitate your mother instead!"

Wherever a Thought Goes, a Chemical Follows

To illustrate this point, imagine that you're walking through a beautiful orchard on a sunny day. As you approach one of the fruit trees, you realize that lemons are the crop in this particular grove. The smell is intoxicating. Because you know that peeling and taking a bite out of one of these lovely yellow lemons would be a very sour experience, you decide you just want to smell one.

So you pluck a lemon from one of the trees and dig your thumbnail into the skin, the sun highlighting a small spray of zest that squirts up. Bringing the lemon to your nose, you breathe in that fresh, elevating, scent-like-no-other and smile with satisfaction.

Later, as you're walking home with sticky hands, you absentmindedly lick your thumb, and are quickly reminded that lemon juice is still on your thumb and it's sour!

Are you salivating, even though there's no real lemon present? This is proof that your thoughts can produce chemical reactions.

Chapter Ten
What a Practitioner Experiences

If you're considering delving into this form of bodywork and becoming a myofascial release therapist, congratulations! I applaud and welcome you.

There will be as much to learn about your own personal growth as there will be to learn about fascia. When you're in service to others, they will reflect back to you your own areas in need of work (especially where your ego or self-love are concerned).

To be your best, understand that you'll need to practice what you preach and keep receiving MFR as much as you're recommending it to others.

I want to set you up to win by sharing a few truths I have learned thanks to time and experience. Let me start with two examples with very different outcomes.

A Tale of Two Outcomes

Kathy

A client whom I'll call Kathy had, for all of her adult life, strongly identified with being a mother and looking pretty. When she came in, referred to me by her chiropractor, she reported pain from an old neck injury.

Even though our intake form asks clients to report any accidents or surgery they've had, I'll ask about it again once we're alone in the treatment room, just in case they didn't want something to be written on paper—or because they might not realize how something that happened a long time ago could be affecting their health now. Also, if the question is posed to clients in a different way, it can jog their memory.

This woman had nothing to add other than what she'd written on her intake form. She explained to me that she had been seeing a massage therapist whom she'd grown "too close" to, and had felt that a change was needed. We began treatment, and I found that her pain was unusually resistant to alleviation.

Kathy told me that the MFR treatments she was now receiving were the only thing making life tolerable for her. After an initial intensive schedule, she chose to continue her treatments once or twice a week, sometimes calling at the last minute, when she felt particularly "tight," to ask me to fit in an extra appointment.

Nearly three months passed before Kathy began to reveal that she was taking antidepressants and had received many corrective surgeries: a nose job, a tummy tuck, a wrist surgery, an ankle surgery, spinal fusion in the lower back, and a facelift.

Eventually Kathy also revealed that she felt so critical about imperfections in her complexion that she would regularly self-administer chemical peels on her face.

When asked by her doctor, "Would you ever harm yourself?" she had replied "No." But she eventually confessed to me that she now realized she'd paid others to do it for her through all of those painful procedures.

During treatment, she spoke of a longing for the days when she was a young mother. Her children, now in adulthood, were not feeling inclined to have children of their own, and this was a source of sadness for Kathy.

But, the more she let go in her body during treatments, the more she was able to let go of her resentment toward her children, husband, parents, and life situation and face the prospect of accepting her current role and finding a new identity in her marriage.

Kathy began to consider returning to work, and over the course of the next year she became very aware that her body had been resisting change. She experienced huge breakthroughs of realization about her mother's expectations of perfection, and began setting up healthy boundaries, while feeling much less triggered, when her parents came to visit.

She started to laugh again and feel more lighthearted during sessions, and eventually brought in her children and parents for treatments as well. With her doctor's supervision, she slowly stopped taking antidepressants. Her husband expressed his gratitude, thanking us for helping his spouse find ease in her body and regain her happiness.

Over the course of that year, Kathy finally transitioned from being a frequent MFR client to seeing clients of her own in her chosen profession. It was heartwarming to see her progress, and to be in her presence as she opened up, expanded, smiled, and laughed.

Then she encountered a place of strong resistance—holding others responsible for how she felt, and avoiding conflict or its resolution—and stopped coming for treatments.

It's not uncommon, in our culture that supports the notion of victimhood, for some clients who have given the practitioner credit for their recovery to eventually shift to blame when encountering a "stuck place" that they're not yet ready to move through.

After that I would sometimes encounter Kathy in town, and it was sad to see that a frown had returned to her face, and to watch her withdraw and retreat within herself, until eventually she and her husband moved back to the place where she had raised her children.

But the point I wish to make is that, in getting to her stuck place, Kathy wasn't wrong. I came to see that this didn't have to *mean* anything. I had to let go and accept that her journey is her own. She wasn't wrong, and I wasn't right.

Brenda

A woman came to see me who, following a blood test, had been told by her doctor that she carried the cancer gene. Her mother had had breast cancer, and so had her sister. The physician's recommendation was that she have a double mastectomy. She quickly agreed.

By the time I saw her, this woman I'm calling Brenda was looking physically great, but I could see by her posture and demeanor that her spirit was very low. As she lay on the table, she began to reveal feelings of grief and depression, as well as overwhelming aches and pains in her body.

The surgical procedure had involved removal of all of her breast tissue and replacement/ reconstruction using fat and fascia from her buttocks. Even though she looked well put together on the outside, on the inside she was suffering from tremendous fascial restriction. In the following months, her treatments involved as much talking, crying, and emotional letting go as they did traction, stretching, and compression.

Once her fascial system began to open and was allowing her more room for movement, Brenda needed to address her alignment issues. Ever since the surgery, her body had been bracing in response to the assault on her fascia and the resulting scars and restrictions.

She was unable to walk in alignment, using her skeletal structure to resist gravity, without recruiting tendons and ligaments in order to remain upright.

Her internally rotated shoulders and the clenching in her buttocks and quadriceps all needed to be addressed so that she could recover, walk upright, and feel her inner vitality once again.

In the course of treatment, it also became clear that she had not been enjoying her chosen career. So what did she do about that? She reeducated herself and began a flourishing career as a myofascial release therapist and alignment expert!

It was so inspiring to see someone get fed up with being sick and tired. Brenda embraced every bit of learning that was available to reverse the downward trend happening in her body, and turned it all around. Her story lends much credibility to her teaching as she shares with others what helped her to recover. "Paying it forward" gives her tremendous job satisfaction now.

The healing journey always continues. Down the road, there will always be opportunities to choose again, because as long as we're alive, we're learning. When we judge ourselves and others, while holding everyone to a standard of perfection, we only perpetuate the internal grip.

The journey continues . . . but only for a lifetime.

I'm Brilliant / I'm Worthless

Doing MFR work gives the practitioner many opportunities to witness clients who are achieving relief from their symptoms of pain. The ego wants to take credit and proclaim, *I'm brilliant! I am so good at this. My clients are lucky to have me.*

However, when progress is slow, or a client begins to feel what might have been deeply buried for years and thinks things are getting worse, or they focus their anger and frustration on the practitioner, accusing you of making them feel something they can't handle, your wounded ego reacts to that as well.

Your ego might say, *I'm worthless at this. I have no business touching people. I should just quit.* When you're attached to the outcome, you can get blown like a leaf from one end of the emotional spectrum to the other—all in the same day.

Dealing with fascia is quite different from dealing with the intellect, which has been rewarded in school and at work for being rational, logical, and linear and for having the right answer. Fascia isn't linear or logical or rational. It is fractal, and it doesn't follow straight lines.

Just going by appearances, one can never know the extent to which other people's lives have caused them to hold and store certain experiences. Accidents, surgeries, injuries, and psychological trauma can all be part of the puzzle. Until I begin treating someone, I know only about those symptoms that the client is aware of. During treatment, the fascial tissue will release what was previously held far from the client's conscious awareness.

What might have started as a stubbed toe when a client was young could have led to a protective holding in the calf and a transfer of weight to the other foot. That might have translated into a shift in the hips that led to a squeezing in the ribs on one side, causing an imbalance in the neck and jaw and resulting in headaches decades later.

But I don't have to know any of that to start treating the individual. I can go by what my hands feel in the body right now.

During treatment, I invite clients to tell me what they're feeling as it occurs. If I'm working on someone's neck and they begin to report an itchy or tingly feeling in their right third toe, I follow their lead and traction the toe for a bit.

When the fascial voice starts talking, we go where it directs us as the story in the body unravels itself.

I can't possibly know about that long-forgotten incident in 1975, nor do I need to. I just follow the client's sensation, knowing that the body on the table will lead me as we gently untangle the snarl.

This work has taught me over and over again not to be attached to a particular outcome. Sometimes my critical mind tells me that, because the client isn't saying anything, this must mean I'm not doing a good job. Then, following the session, the client reports that he was seeing colors behind his closed eyes and remembering things long forgotten from childhood, or that he had sunk more deeply into relaxation than he'd been able to do in ten years.

As my mentor, John Barnes, so wisely counseled, "The worst that can happen is nothing," and I must sometimes remind myself of that so I can let my hands and the client's fascia lead.

The Best Giver Is a Good Receiver

For me, the best reminder happens when I receive my own MFR treatments. By regularly receiving myofascial release, I remain in touch with what my clients are experiencing. What I can learn to allow and let go of in my own body helps me to facilitate the same allowing and release for others.

Each client has a different path, and it is through their allowing, awareness, and letting go that clients navigate their way out of pain. If I provide the time, place, teaching, and touch for this, my own intellect doesn't have to get involved. My hands know what to do.

Here in Ojai, Teresa Jayne is my craniosacral therapist, and a mentor who taught me a method of using my body as a channel of energy so that I can facilitate the movement of others' energy without it getting hung up in me.

When I teach myofascial release to future practitioners, I highly recommend that my students learn this technique that Teresa calls "Earth Energy Healing." I want them to enjoy their work and continue to do so for years to come, avoiding the burnout so common to traditional massage therapists.

Chapter Eleven
Life in a Massage Mill

For a number of years, I worked in massage mills. I call them this even though they were quite fancy—even exquisite—places. Where management's attitude toward employees was concerned, it was plain to see that their business model was designed around money, not humans. The following was my experience.

So that the company didn't have to take responsibility as an employer, a massage therapist was considered to be an independent contractor. Legally, that should mean that you could set your own fees, show up when they had work for you, bill them, and account for your own taxes, health insurance, savings, etc.

In reality, they required you to agree to a work schedule and to clock in and sit there whether they had work for you or not. No clients, no money.

Weekly staff meetings were mandatory whether these took place during your shift or not; they would pay you minimum wage to attend. Working on weekends and holidays was compulsory.

An Abysmal Pay Scale

The mill collected all fees and kept all tips (cash included), promising to take out taxes and to write employees a paycheck every two weeks. Records were kept and reprimands given, and any raises were based on the number of years the employee had worked there.

Where the facility would charge $125 for a Swedish massage, we would start out making $29, with the hope of working our way all the way to the top of the scale, after six years of employment, to a whopping $46 per hour.

Any request for a weekend or holiday off had to be submitted to the administration thirty days in advance, with no guarantee that our request would be granted. Uniforms were required, along with a strict dress code.

An additional hoop to jump through was added when the facility wanted bragging rights about the skill level of their massage therapists. They required that we obtain national certification (a $250 fee, borne by us, and a rigorous 125-question written exam that therapists agonized over and studied for months to pass). Without this certification, we would never make more than $39 an hour.

When we were first employed, extensive training was required, during which time we were compensated with the minimum wage.

Much time was spent teaching us how to do the "signature" treatments that included salt scrubs, aromatherapy, and hot towels. (We needed to wear fire safety gloves when we pulled those towels from the scalding water, and had to be careful not to reach so deeply as to let the water run down into the gloves).

We were also versed in specific guidelines for how to interact with the clients as defined by the American Automobile Association for their coveted Diamond Ratings. To quote AAA: "Establishments must consistently reflect upscale and extraordinary characteristics (respectively) in both physical attributes and level of guest services."

Spa Doublespeak

Each patron was to be called a guest. We were instructed never to turn our back to guests or walk ahead of them, which involved some fancy footwork at times, when a guest didn't know that you were trying to avoid having her see your back.

When approached by guests asking to be directed to some part of the facility, strict guidelines prevented me from simply pointing out the desired locale and called for me to walk there with them. I found it quietly hilarious when they would be waiting for me to lead the way while I was trying to encourage them to walk beside me instead of behind me. This led to some awkward dance moves that I eventually learned to perfect.

Emphasis was placed on the word "upsell"—coined to denote the skill of mentioning other services of which the guests must certainly avail themselves.

For instance, "After you've finished washing away the dead skin cells following your salt scrub, you'll thank yourself for taking advantage of our heated sauna! Also, you'll be excited to know that you can purchase the signature moisturizing cream we used at the end of your pampering. It's conveniently available in the salon lobby, and I can easily add it to your receipt."

Another term I'd never heard before was *going forward*, used by administration as a nice way to emphasize that you'd screwed up. It was a veiled threat, meant to imply "Don't ever let it happen again." In other words, "Going forward, an error of this nature will be met with immediate dismissal."

We were never to say the word "no" (not even "no problem"), and were encouraged to use words like "certainly," "my pleasure," "perfect," and "yes." This might explain why, if you've ever called to schedule such a treatment, the "hospitality staff" has responded over and over again in hyperbole.

You: "I'd like to schedule a treatment."

Phone personality: "Awesome. Do you know what you would like, or can I share the details of what we have to offer?"

You: "I'd like a one-hour Swedish massage, please."

Phone personality: "Excellent. It sounds like our 50-minute Classic Swedish Massage would be perfect for you. For your convenience, I can take your payment information now so you don't have to hassle with that after you've had your treatment and you want to enjoy your bliss."

You: "Okay. It's a Visa."

Phone personality: "Perfect. Any time you're ready, I can enter your information."

After the information is shared, there are more exclamations of "Fantastic!" and "Super!" and "Amazing!" before you're let off the line.

Win-Lose Situations

One was required to massage five guests in a row, take an hour break, and see one more guest before clocking out. Or vice versa: clock in, do one massage, take an hour break, do five more, and then clock out.

Each massage was to start promptly on the hour and end ten minutes before the next hour. (Innumerable clients noticed the time with a glance, a comment of "Is that it?" or a request that you address just one more area of need: "Can you do a little more on my feet"? This clearly communicated that, if you wanted a good tip, you would give them a full hour of massage.

During that precious ten-minute gap, you were to wait for the client to get dressed and come out of the room, present them with a cup of spa water with cucumber and lemon, up-sell the other treatments and spa facilities, say the client's name three times, politely hand them an evaluation card, and walk them back to the locker rooms.

Then you were to return to the treatment room, remove the used sheets, replace them and return the room to pristine condition.

Next, you needed to check the computer in the break room to see your next room assignment and client, fill out their name on an evaluation card, make sure the new room was in perfect order, and then retrieve your next guest from the waiting lounge while appearing sweat-free and calm.

As I mentioned, part of the protocol when wrapping up a guest interaction after a massage was to hand the patron an evaluation card with your name on it. It felt like begging for praise, but it was also a vehicle for criticism that made us cringe, since there were so many variables that we couldn't control.

One enterprise that employed me had an audible rat problem in the ceiling, as well as antiquated heating and air conditioning. We massage therapists never knew if we would be sweltering or shivering in those rooms, but we did know that we'd hear about it via the tip and on those evaluation cards.

At the mills, an awkward situation would often occur. The facilities agreed never to schedule you with back-to-back deep tissue massages or more than two deep tissue massages a day. But a guest might schedule the least expensive Swedish massage and then, after lying on the table for the first few strokes, say, "You can go much deeper than that. I have a high pain tolerance."

Well now, that would be a more expensive Deep Tissue massage. Remember, you're working for that 20 percent tip that could double what you're getting paid for that hour. And you're forbidden to say no to a guest.

Even though the deep tissue massage is more expensive, you won't be paid more; it will just increase your potential tip. Do you tell the client, "Fantastic—that will mean an increase in the price of the treatment; if you wish, I'll be happy to add that to your receipt," or do you simply do as you're asked, without discussion?

I found out the hard way, with a nasty comment on the evaluation card and a reprimand from the manager, that the only acceptable answer to give was, "Certainly." You just did it, hoping the guest would reward you with a better tip for being so pleasing and agreeable.

Before I go on, let me acknowledge that I know I'm whining in this chapter. So let me put a spin on it and call it "describing." Most people don't know the eye-opening stuff that goes on behind the scenes at luxurious spas, and I think they should. That being said, there's more.

Why We Stayed

As I write this, I'm still amazed at what was asked of us as massage therapists, and that we pulled it off. We developed the kind of camaraderie that happens in groups of people who have gone through some kind of hellish experience together.

There were times of feast and times of famine. During the down times, we would flirt, tell jokes, play games, massage each other, make up arguments, and—most of all—complain.

Despite everything, though, we actually did believe we were lucky to work there.

The administration never failed to let us know that many other massage therapists would be happy to take our place, so the kind of complaining we did was akin to that of someone bemoaning a bad relationship.

As time went on, a codependent bond was formed. Believing there was no other choice, and hiding from ourselves the truth about the "victim points" we earned (and enjoyed when bragging to others about how abused we were), we stayed on.

What made the massage mill a seemingly attractive alternative to starting a private practice was the challenge of building one's own client base. It doesn't happen overnight, and many really good therapists give up early on because (1) they don't have an alternative income stream to support them while they build their practice, (2) they don't have the skill, patience, or budget to do the marketing necessary to generate clientele, or (3) they measure their value based on the limited number of clients they have starting out and get discouraged.

These massage mills had a big local presence, and advertised well to their high-end clientele. They had huge marketing budgets, and targeted the rich and famous. This meant that occasionally one would get to work on a famous person.

Because we signed confidentiality agreements, I can't name names, but it felt good to respect the privacy of celebrities and give them a chance to relax, relieved of their own fame for a while. In fact, I know that in their private moments they complained about the life they had chosen in the same way that we did.

How I Found Out What Doesn't Work

One February day, I happened to have done *six* deep-tissue massages, and my left shoulder was screaming by the end of my shift. At that time I didn't know any better so when I got home I put an ice pack on it. When I got up early the next morning, my shoulder still felt quite painful.

One of my extra duties was to open the facility each morning. I was usually the only person there for an hour, and I enjoyed the quiet and felt a sense of pride in making the place guest-ready.

That morning, I was really worried that if I did any massage I'd be in a lot of pain. Once you start a massage, there's no taking a break. You engage with that person's body and stay engaged with it for the full time until you're done.

I tried to get hold of the manager, to let her know that I needed a replacement. When she called me back, none too happy at that early hour, I told her about the day before and that I was scheduled with a guest for a deep tissue massage first thing that morning.

Her advice to me was, "Do the best you can." She knew it would be hard to find a replacement right away, and was hoping I could just get through this one till other therapists arrived who could take the rest of my appointments.

I said I would try, and I did. I carried out that one further deep massage, and thus began my adventure into the world of workers' compensation insurance.

That afternoon, the X-rays showed a partial tear in the rotator cuff of my left shoulder.

During the next few weeks, I was treated to hours of waiting in doctors' offices, and repeated interrogation as to how this might have happened.

"When did you first notice the symptoms?" I was asked, and, "What might you have done at home that could have caused this injury?"

During this time the manager called me and said that, had she known just how much I was hurting, she would never have asked me to do the massage that morning. It's likely that she was legally required to have that conversation on record in her files.

This adventure really fed my belief in my own victimhood. It hurt. I couldn't work. So I thought I had to jump through their hoops and agree to all the recommended treatments. I'm grateful that I can now see how this was showing me what did *not* work to heal my shoulder, and leading me to search for what *did*.

One part of my medical "vacation" was very interesting. When the workers' comp doctor arrived in the exam room two hours after my scheduled appointment, he said that he had looked at the X-rays and they showed a one-inch bone fragment in my shoulder.

He opined that this could not have occurred from doing massages, and interrogated me further, convinced (and working to convince *me*) that I must have done something dramatic on my own time to create such an injury.

I had always wondered what it would be like to be accused of a crime one didn't commit, and it felt like this was the moment I was going to find out.

I stared.

He stared.

I said, "Are you kidding me?"

He stared.

I said, "I don't know what to tell you. I know where I was and what I did, and if you're telling me that I have a one-inch bone fragment floating around in my shoulder, I'm very alarmed that something like that could have happened so easily without my knowing it. Is it an indication of a bigger problem?"

Finally he referred me to an orthopedic specialist.

The specialist showed me the X-rays, and informed me that what the other physician had seen as a bone fragment was a calcification in my deltoid muscle. I saw it. It was on the outside of my upper arm muscle, and was about the size and shape of an almond.

The fellow meant to be reassuring as he told me that this was just a calcification of the fascial tissue from overuse (known as calcific tendonitis), and had nothing to do with the injury to my rotator cuff. He said that many people have one of these calcifications and don't even know about it, unless an X-ray for something else happens to reveal it.

Because the rotator cuff tear was only partial and didn't warrant surgery, he suggested a cortisone injection for the pain. He advised me that this brought immediate relief to most patients but could erode the connective tissue, so I would be allowed only one.

The injection hurt like hell, and did nothing to alleviate the pain.

In the meantime, I went through my days trying not to move my left shoulder. When I would forget and try to unscrew a lid or reach up to a shelf, an involuntary yelp would escape my lips. I would try to stop my eyes from watering with pain and self-pity, so the kids wouldn't get upset. When the pain overcame me, I'd shout out, "I'm okay!" just as fast as I could.

Physical therapy was next. If I didn't comply and keep the appointments, workers' comp would dismiss me as noncompliant and I'd be stuck footing the bill for everything accumulated to that point . . . while still unable to work. So off I trotted to my scheduled appointments.

These also involved a lot of waiting. When the PT came into the exam room, he was rough and gruff and often began manhandling me with no preamble or explanation. Over my clothing, he would do something like massage, and the movements were quick and included a lot of deep repetitive squeezing.

I never let him see me cry. He would put me through some range-of-motion testing and show me some exercises to do that were designed to strengthen the muscles but primarily just aggravated the ache. Afterward he would show me a circuit of weight machines and leave me on my own to do repetitions of arm pulldowns and bicep curls.

After four or five of those visits, I was sent on to see the occupational therapist. The OT was a nice woman who would line up several of us at a long table that was akin to a bar, where she was like the bartender.

Sitting in her chair, she would roll up and down the length of the table full of patients and give us various games to do with our hands, like pulling rubber bands and squeezing rubber balls. My favorite part was when she would smooth an icy-hot type of lotion on my arm and wrap it in a hot towel for a while.

In the back of my mind I knew that, when all was said and done, I was going to make a beeline to a myofascial release therapist. I was hoping to interrupt the holding patterns that were developing in all the areas around the pain in my shoulder.

Once all the various physical treatments were completed, I was released, and what I was released to was about the same amount of pain I'd had going in. I was learning to live with it and to compensate. Because I was still in no shape to return to work, my employers agreed to let me be an on-call therapist on the weekends. Over the next few months they called me once or twice, but I never felt ready to jump back in and do twelve massages in two days.

I began paying out-of-pocket from my savings to see a wonderful MFR therapist once a week. Her work increased my range of motion and brought great relief to the holding in my neck, chest, shoulder blades, back, and arm.

A Blessing in Disguise

During one of my visits with the MFR therapist, she told me about an exercise studio that had asked her to rent a room and offer myofascial release there. She had turned them down because she was happy staying right where she was, but she asked if I thought I might be able to do that kind of work and get away from the massage mill.

I loved doing MFR, and missed the days when I wasn't someone's employee. I knew it had been much easier on my body, and I really didn't want to go back to doing deep tissue massage because it was so taxing, and yet not as therapeutically beneficial as myofascial release.

After calling to set up an interview, I was greeted by a most engaging, intelligent, energetic, and authentic young woman. She completely understood the value of myofascial release, and said she wasn't going to offer the treatment room for rent to anyone else because she was so confident that MFR was what she wanted as a complement to the alignment work she was doing with her clients.

I was impressed and pleased. The rent was reasonable, because I would be sharing the room with a massage therapist who was already doing Swedish massage there three days a week.

Here is the ugly truth of what I was thinking while going into this arrangement. I thought the young woman was some sort of aerobics instructor, and that I was doing her a favor. I thought that, because I understood fascia, my knowledge was superior to hers. I thought that, once she experienced my work, I'd be able to teach her about it, raise her to my level, and maybe even influence her to change her perspective about exercise.

For months, on my way to the treatment room to give MFR sessions I walked past classes this woman was teaching, with no thought of ever joining in.

She encouraged her students to make appointments with me, and I scheduled them to see me without regard to the times that her classes were in session.

I thought that what the clients would receive from me would be so much more valuable than any exercise class.

I was annoyed by the proximity of the exercise space to my treatment room. This woman had trained others to teach for her, and one of the teachers had a distractingly piercing voice. I couldn't wait to give that one a treatment and calm her down.

In short, I was being an idiot.

The owner expressed concern for my shoulder injury, and offered, even though she was very busy, to trade one of her private instruction sessions in return for a myofascial release treatment from me. *Aha! My chance to blow her mind.*

She received. She loved it. I then received an alignment evaluation from a student that the owner was training. She stood close by, giving her student some hints and making notes on a check sheet.

I didn't tell the student about my injury, because I wasn't sure if I was supposed to let her figure out my area of weakness on her own. With prompting from her teacher, she put me into a position to externally rotate my shoulders with gentle traction, and the tears started to roll down my cheeks.

I breathed. I shook. The owner kept reassuring me that this was making things better, not worse. I didn't believe her, and I realized that my tears were not so much from pain as from anger at the massage mill that had pushed me to work till I "broke."

When the session was over, I felt *life* ooze back into my shoulder and arm.

That night, the pain that had become so familiar did not return. My evaluator and her mentor had given me two key exercises to do that were nothing like the ones I'd been given by the PT or OT. *And every single time I did them, I felt better.*

I became a devoted attendee of all the young woman's classes, and eventually earned certification to teach the program she had developed.

Through all my years of practice as a massage therapist, I knew that I could help folks feel better. I just didn't know how to keep them from coming back over and over again with the same symptoms.

That might sound odd: keep them from coming back? Isn't the idea to keep them coming back?

No. Healing is the idea.

What this woman taught me was a missing piece that complemented my practice and satisfied my desire to help people find long-term relief. It provided a way to teach clients how patterns of holding in the fascia become ingrained with habitual misalignment, and how they could sustain the progress they gained from treatment.

In particular, I learned that prolonged *sitting* is a major culprit in causing the common diseases thought to be associated with aging, such as joint pain, heart and lung disease, and pelvic and digestive disorders, to name just a few.

That fateful alignment evaluation in 2007 turned out to play a major part in leading me to where I am today. With my partner, Joe Cocke, I co-own a thriving business in Ojai, California, where we serve our community by showing them that aging needn't mean inevitable decrepitude. At Sanctuary, we combine the modalities of MFR and alignment within our own True Body™ system.

This has proven to be an especially opportune time to serve the population of aging baby boomers who never have settled for the status quo. They vote with their feet, often only after having exhausted all the treatments still being recommended by Western medicine. The number of letters after my name matters less to my fellow boomers than how they feel after receiving treatment and learning to sustain their progress.

People come to the Sanctuary offices in great numbers because we help them to feel better, and they leave empowered with tools to help them maintain ease in their body, without dependence on anyone or anything but themselves.

Chapter Twelve
Who's Healing Whom?

In the scenario where someone comes to me for a treatment and they're undressed and lying on a table under a sheet looking up at me, I used to think that made me the giver, and therefore they were the receiver.

This must mean that they have questions and I have the answers, I thought.

It now sounds so arrogant and judgmental when I follow these thought patterns to the bottom.

That must mean that I'm superior and they're inferior.

Since I'm the one who's healing them, I should call myself a healer.

This duality thinking could get even worse.

I'm up; they're down.

I'm good; they're bad.

They're broken, and I must fix them.

They must be wrong, and I must be right.

It can be nauseating for me to realize my own former underlying attitudes, unconscious and unspoken.

Through the years, it began to dawn on me that everyone is my teacher. My clients allow me to express my soul's desire to serve. Without them, I'd be thwarted. And it is by exploring the buried experiences in my own body through myofascial release that I learn how to guide my clients in doing the same.

This has also brought home to me the realization that part of my job is to "clean my own house." In other words, thank you, Mom and Dad and everyone else, for my childhood of contrasts that has helped highlight for me, many times over, who I am not and where I need to grow and heal.

My Cycles of Learning

Each spiral of my personal journey seems to follow these steps:

1. A huge problem
2. Extreme discomfort
3. Fear
4. Avoidance
5. The problem gets bigger
6. Suppressed anger
7. A huge, indelicate blowup
8. My worst fears realized

9. The realization of my part in creating it all
10. My humble admission of responsibility
11. Circumstances way better than before

That sequence happened for each one of about a thousand growth experiences before I began to notice a pattern. With this realization, I have now gingerly begun experimenting with skipping Steps 4 through 8.

One day I was in conflict with someone where I worked. A client I was scheduled to see happened to be the mother of the person I was having the conflict with. When she arrived, I thought I would just put up a wall and keep it to myself. But when the mother innocently asked how things were going, I started to cry.

I wasn't free to explain the details of my upset. I apologized, and the tears kept coming. I eventually found myself sitting on the floor, tissues in both hands, heaving sobs of sweet release.

Then I wanted to leave the room. I felt humiliated by my inappropriateness and lack of control, and really wanted to run. But the woman wouldn't let me go. Her compassion and ability to quietly hold space allowed me to empty myself of the physical holding and then proceed with a treatment that was so tender, real, and heartfelt that I remember it to this day.

I'm not suggesting that this is a helpful therapeutic method. (I was lucky that the mother was so compassionate and understanding.) But hiding your humanity isn't the goal, either. What I'm saying is that the therapeutic road isn't a one-way street.

The Healing Exchange

For me, the term "healer" brings up images of a preacher in a tent bilking people out of their money by getting them emotionally worked up into thinking he was chosen by God to get rid of their pain—if they only have enough faith and sufficient dough-re-mi.

So I don't refer to myself as a healer. My clients' fascia, chemistry, intellect, and feelings are entirely theirs. Healing happens within them, and it happens because they allow it. I prefer to see my role as that of a facilitator.

Try going into a room where you're alone with someone for an hour or more and just keeping yourself to yourself.

Better yet, try not to be moved when a person allows herself to feel, physically and emotionally, what has been buried deep inside her, taking up space and energy, since she was pulled from a crumpled taxi twenty-five years ago with a broken pelvis, severe lacerations, and head trauma.

I tried. I used to believe that it was my professional responsibility to not be moved. Yet I would notice myself being irritable and stiff after each session. The effect of all that emotional and physical resistance was eventually dysfunctional.

Once I admitted that it did affect me, and dared to express my authentic responses during treatments, I saw that I was able to let go of the resistance within me to whatever important buried feelings my clients might be moving through.

If *my* emotions were making *me* uncomfortable, I could only imagine how clients on the table must have been feeling about their own. I began to notice (usually in retrospect) that, when I was reluctant to face and deal with some particular issue in my life, I would attract clients who were demonstrating the same resistance.

A natural selection began to occur. When I would move through something and experience personal growth, those clients who weren't ready in that area of growth would naturally drift away, while others who were willing to face those issues started showing up. Healing could occur because I had allowed it in *me*, and then I knew that it was possible for *them*.

Energies and Frequencies

The unseen can be measured. Here's where my study of audiology comes in handy. Energy can be measured in waves. How high the wave goes is called the amplitude. How often the wave repeats is the frequency. This creates a signature vibration that can be measured. Everyone's body has vibrational frequencies that can be measured from moment to moment, and different parts of the body will vibrate at different rates, depending on the local tissue density.

Energy constantly moves out and in. Think about how, when you drop a pebble into a pond, a series of circlets goes outward. Meanwhile, under the water's surface, those circlets are returning to the exact spot where you dropped in the pebble.

In electromagnetic force, the out-moving flow of those circlets is electric energy and the inward-moving flow is magnetic energy. All matter emits a measurable electromagnetic frequency. At a lower vibration, things move slowly—like walking through deep water. At a higher frequency, movement is quickened and easy.

When vibrational energies match, they draw in more of the same vibrational frequency and are amplified (crystals are used this way in radio transmissions). When they don't match, the higher frequency serves to increase the rate of the lower frequency.

Think of energy as being of two distinct types: force and flow. Flow energy is a vibrational match to the frequency of love. Force is a vibrational match to the frequency of fear. A great resource for this information is the book *Power vs. Force: The Hidden Determinants of Human Behavior* by David R. Hawkins, MD, PhD. It provides a chart showing the measurements of human emotions using muscle testing.

This explains how we attract clients and the influence we wield, as well as the importance of intentionally keeping our own frequency high. When our bodies are dense with restriction and resistance, our tissues can't respond to movement with ease. And this is why I find it just as important for me to receive this mfr work frequently as it is to provide it.

When pressure is applied to certain kinds of material (such as crystals, some ceramics, and biological matter such as bone, dna, and various proteins) an electrical charge is generated.

To read an article that explains very well the role of piezoelectricity in bodywork, you can either go online to Wikipedia and search for "Piezoelectricity" or scan this QR code to get to the same page:

The importance of this scientific principle to myofascial release is that, when pressure is applied by the therapist at a 45 degree angle, it changes the shape of the client's body, deforming the collagen molecules and generating piezoelectricity, thus increasing the negative electric charge of the collagen molecules. This increases the growth and regeneration of tissue.

The therapist is causing a change in the electromagnetic field of the client. And not only is there a change in the tissue being touched, but a reciprocal effect occurs in the hands and arms of the person applying the touch.

If I apply techniques of myofascial release to your body, I'm also experiencing electrical responses from you. It's not a one-way street. We are affecting each other, and this effect is not a subjective observation but objective, and scientifically quantifiable in tens to hundreds of microwatts.

MFR treatments help to bring the body into vibrational coherence by easing areas of physical resistance. With fewer snarls and more light flowing through the microtubules, there are fewer areas where the flow of energy is slowed. The body's frequency can then become consistent throughout. In other words, we're better conductors of energy when we have fewer kinks in our pipes.

Chapter Thirteen
A Fascia Q&A

Is foam rolling like myofascial release?

No it's not, although this is a common misconception. MFR displaces the skin to separate it from the layers of superficial fascia, whereas foam rolling crushes together the skin and fascial layers.

Instead of foam rollers, I recommend using various sizes of therapy balls, which have less resistance and allow 360 degrees of sinking in. Foam rollers are too hard, and the way in which they're used doesn't cause a displacement of fascia but creates a crushing effect on all the tissues a roller is applied to.

A popular fad among runners is to use a foam roller to try to release the iliotibial band, a tight strip of muscle on the outer thigh. In positioning himself on the roller, a runner will bear most of his body weight on one elbow.

As he shifts up and down the side of one thigh on the roller while his shoulder compensates for the movement, he'll likely be unaware of the alignment that would be needed to ensure that his shoulder isn't incurring damage from this. Meanwhile he's holding a belief that the pain of all this is somehow working to his benefit.

The speed at which he does this, and the override of his internal monitoring system that's telling him it hurts, combine with the fact that the roller isn't displacing the fascia under the skin but rather crushing the skin and fascia together. So foam rolling is not like myofascial release, as it creates bracing, micro-tears in the fascia, and possible adhesions. All these can only lead to a more limited range of motion.

The method of self-myofascial release that I teach requires the use of dense therapy balls in varying sizes, and involves waiting in each spot for 90 to 120 seconds of release to every area of the body. Students notice the amount of resistance they find when they first lie on the ball, and are asked to imagine their fascia softening and melting as though they're absorbing the ball into their body—rather than punishing their body for misbehaving with an aggressive attitude of "no pain, no gain" as they would aggressively grind down on a foam roller.

In doing self-MFR, we allow our intuition to guide us to where the body is calling for the ball to be placed next. We do not "spot clean" the body by following a systematic routine, but follow what comes into our awareness as the lines of fascia running throughout the body begin to tell the story of where the patterns of holding are connected.

In a workshop of a hundred or more people, the energy of the group strongly contributes to finding breakthroughs in areas of the body that have for years contained painful holding patterns. The experience of light and lightness in the body sends folks away with a joyful euphoria not often seen on the faces of runners.

How does chiropractic adjustment relate to MFR?

A "tent" analogy really helps to explain the role of chiropractic work as it relates to myofascial release. Conjure any memory you might have of an old-fashioned tent with a central tent pole. We'll compare that tent pole to your spine.

When attempting to raise a tent like that, we used to start with the central pole and then use guy wires (tensioned cables designed to add stability to a free-standing structure) evenly around the sides to help the pole remain straight. If any of those guy wires were off, it didn't matter how many times you pushed or pulled on the center pole, the tent pole wouldn't stay straight if the guy wires were exerting forces in other directions.

Comparing the guy wires to fascial restriction explains the benefit of having an MFR treatment before a chiropractic adjustment, and shows why the adjustment is then more likely to have lasting effects. That is to say, if you have a holding pattern in your shoulder and a lot of discomfort in your neck, it's no use trying to adjust the spine without adjusting the shoulder's holding pattern, because the holding pattern in the shoulder will keep pulling the spine out of alignment. The tension on the "guy wire" needs to be loosened in order for the spine to stay in alignment.

The reason chiropractic adjustment doesn't help to release fascial restriction is because a characteristic function of fascia is protection. It braces in response to sudden movement, so if you approach it with a mobilization technique using force or speed, it will simply resist with all the strength it can muster, which can be as much as two thousand pounds of tensile strength.

How does an MFR treatment compare to getting a massage?

Receiving myofascial release is not at all like getting a massage. Because in MFR traction on the skin is needed, no oil is used; this is why we request that no morning moisturizer be applied on the day of treatment. Swedish massage uses petrissage (squeezing) and effleurage (sweeping) motions to glide over the skin, aided by lotion or oil. This makes it impossible to engage the superficial fascial layer with any kind of traction.

The MFR approach is to, once gaining traction on the skin, press in the direction of ease and wait there for ninety seconds to five minutes, giving the body the chance it needs to soften and let the fascia "melt," letting go of the holding and restriction.

Studies show that engaging with a fascial restriction for five minutes stimulates a secretion of interleukin 8 (IL-8), an anti-inflammatory protein naturally produced by the body. Most massage treatments move too quickly and don't allow for the release that comes with sustained traction.

"Mall massage" businesses in increasing numbers are inviting us to lie down fully clothed and receive a variation of shiatsu massage.

This doesn't allow the therapist to engage the skin at all. He or she is engaging the fabric of your clothing, and the most that can be achieved is compression, which is the intended style of shiatsu but not the aim of myofascial release.

This would be a good time to make the distinction between myofascial release and "trigger points"—defined, in massage, as tight areas within muscle tissue that cause pain in other parts of the body. In MFR, we know when we find an especially sore spot that fascial restriction is inhibiting the flow of blood and lymph through that area. Applying fingertip pressure to the area, as massage therapists are taught to do, misses the understanding that a "trigger point" is only a symptom.

The sore area is part of a fascial web. Limb traction near the area, or displacing the skin above the area, can do more to release the restriction and restore flow than having someone just press straight downward onto tissues that are already sticking together, thereby exacerbating a spot that's already sore and creating no more space for flow.

Is there a pill for fascial restriction?

If a fire alarm were going off in your house, would you prefer that the firemen rush in and put out the fire, or that they simply turn off the alarm and walk away?

This seems like a no-brainer, right? But, too often, people take a pill that serves only to turn off an alarm, not to resolve the bodily problem that's bothering them.

A physical symptom such as pain, swelling and inflammation, a limited range of motion, or poor digestion and elimination is an alarm. It's telling you that you have a problem in your body that needs to be addressed.

When you go to the doctor, he or she will likely prescribe medication. The drugs of choice for fascial pain are NSAIDS (refer to Chapter Six regarding their adverse effects on fascia), muscle relaxers, corticosteroids, and opioids. You may then get relief from some of your symptoms, but you haven't yet addressed the reason that your body is trying to get your attention in the first place. This is the equivalent of turning off the alarm instead of putting out the fire. And evidence keeps emerging that, over time, these actually worsen the pain and create more problems than they solve.

I have a diagnosis, but could my symptoms actually be caused by fascial restriction?

Without an understanding of fascia and its function, doctors are often baffled as to the origin of a disease process or its solution. They apply the term *idiopathic origin*, meaning that they don't know how or why it started. And these "diseases" sometimes resolve themselves for reasons that doctors can't explain.

The origins of many diagnosed ills can be known if one understands the effects of fascial holding patterns. In fibromyalgia, infertility, TMJ syndrome, plantar fasciitis, high blood pressure, trigeminal neuralgia syndrome, pelvic floor dysfunction, thoracic outlet syndrome, degenerative disc disease, etc., what you're dealing with is a manifestation of a lifetime of fight-or-flight response.

For a view of the many disorders associated with fascia, you can go online to Wikipedia and search for "Disorders of Fascia" or scan this QR code:

Without an understanding of connective tissue, physicians are left guessing at the origin and experimenting with solutions. My experience as a doctor's wife showed me that physicians really do want to help, but they get frustrated when someone keeps returning with the same complaint. It causes them to go outside the scope of their training and try outlandish things.

I saw one MFR client whose doctor had proposed that, to solve the chronic hip pain on one side of her body, they sever her psoas muscle on that side.

Trigeminal neuralgia, which causes intractable shooting pains in the face, used to also be called "suicide disease." This diagnosis is most common among females over the age of fifty, and anti-seizure medication is the preferred prescription, usually followed by muscle relaxers and antidepressants. The treatment is generally expected to be continued for years.

Yet the goal is to heal, right?

If I were a doctor, before I sent someone out of my office with a prescription for an anti-seizure medication—the side effects of which could make her a frequent return visitor—I'd much rather take a less dramatic approach and see what might happen with gentle traction, compression, and emotional release.

How does fascia affect my heart?

Constricted fascia plays a large role in creating high blood pressure. If you picture a balloon that's been inflated inside a fishnet stocking, with the fishnet being progressively squeezed and twisted, you can see why your heart will eventually have a harder time pumping blood into that balloon as the pressure on its outside keeps being increased.

Stretching and receiving MFR is far better for your heart than a heavy cardio workout, because it *reduces* the resistance your heart must work against. You're much better off *taking the pressure off the balloon* than making the heart pump harder.

A healthy venous system naturally expands in response to the kind of intermittent squeezing produced by active physical movement. In contrast, fascial holding patterns create a constant, static pressure. In other words, a pressure that never lets up.

When the holding patterns in your fascia are never interrupted, it leaves no room for your veins to expand and consequently, there's less and less room for blood circulation. Your blood vessels atrophy and are reabsorbed until your circulatory system can barely supply blood to anything beyond your torso.

If you have a sedentary job, and head out to the gym for a one-hour heavy cardio workout after a day of scarcely interrupted sitting, your body will release a stress hormone (cortisol) in response to your heart being asked to pump so hard into a tight fascial system.

Often the people who think they're doing a good thing for their body by exercising don't realize that, while their doctor may have told them to diet and exercise, he or she didn't direct them as to *what* diet or *what* exercise to pursue—probably because these are not areas within the physician's expertise.

Much has been researched and published regarding the "yo-yo" effects of dieting. Doctors who understand that varied movement and healthful eating habits support all physical systems would rather use such prescriptive words as "good nutrition and whole-body movement throughout the day."

Is myofascial release like Rolfing, and is it supposed to hurt?

Ida Rolf had the right idea; she knew that fascial restriction was a problem. Yet she taught her Rolfing practitioners to exert a great amount of force to interrupt fascial patterns and make them let go. When patients would scream in pain, they were encouraged to breathe through it.

The tensile strength of fascia can resist two thousand pounds of pressure. The goal of MFR is to avoid causing any more bracing in a client's body; they've had enough practice doing that. The challenge is to find our way "in" by finding the direction of ease.

We have no way of knowing where the initial bracing began. We allow our hands to "ask questions" into a client's body, without requiring the client to "give in." By pressing or pulling in the direction of ease until we meet resistance, and then going only to the point just before the body begins to brace, what we offer is not a command but an invitation to let go.

With sustained traction or compression, we eventually feel a slight give, like the softening of clay. When we wait in that way for the body to give its permission, the person on the table is able to sink into much deeper layers than would be possible if he or she were bracing against pain. Clients will still feel sensation, and still make sounds in response. But, when they do, we want those sounds to be from feeling emotions and letting go, not from pain.

Are there side effects?

We notice some really interesting side effects in many people following treatment. Clients commonly report urinating a great deal after a session. They report being very thirsty after a session. They report having a beer, a glass of wine, or a cup of coffee after a session and being thrown for a loop. Because fascia is super-absorbent when its restrictions have been eased, the effects of alcohol and caffeine can be multiplied post-treatment.

As the body starts to clear its clutter, people become intolerant of clutter elsewhere in their lives. They report cleaning out a junk drawer at home, or ask if the treatment could be the reason they went home and were able to resolve a longstanding difference with a loved one.

Clients will ask if it's normal for them to feel particularly childish, loving, emotional, or exhausted post-treatment. The answer is yes. Along with the feeling of lightness and more space in the body comes a return to one's more authentic, vulnerable, joyful self. Need I say that this is in quite some contrast to the side effects listed on commercials for prescription meds?

The Buddha is quoted as saying, "The mind talks; the body knows." In the phenomenon known as a *healing crisis*, your body has held its encapsulated cocktails of chemistry for years. As it begins to tell the truth it never had a chance to tell before, a number of things can happen.

You might experience fever, fatigue, headache, congestion, insomnia, restlessness, body aches, or emotional upheaval. Basically, you might revisit the suppressed feelings of a lifetime.

Have you ever had a coffee habit and quit cold turkey? Then you know the kind of headache that even such a mini healing crisis can produce. When some clients experience the uncomfortable phase of healing, that's when things can become the most tenuous.

When there's something you've been trying your whole life *not* to feel, it can make you wonder why you're doing this.

The increased physical sensation or the flooding of an emotional dam can cause you to weigh the prices and payoffs of treatment. This can be the point at which a client will say, "I think I'm coming down with something. I should cancel my appointment." This reaction isn't my favorite thing, because it's like starting a course of antibiotics and not finishing it. It isn't fun for you to be left in some miserable, achy, emotional state for weeks on end.

The idea is to move through the healing crisis as quickly as you can and not stay suspended in that limbo. You're not coming down with something; you're letting go of something you already have.

This is exactly the time that I want a client to keep coming in, so we can move through that layer and not leave them feeling that way for any extended period of time. The only way out is through, and the only way through is to let your body release what it has held for years.

An enormous element of *trust* comes into play in this therapeutic exchange. Your MFR therapist wants to get in there with you and guide you through so that you don't have to keep revisiting this phase. You'll be surprised at how quickly you can move through the yucky spots as you continue treatment.

You're always free to decide whether the possibility of a fascial freedom that you aren't even sure exists is worth the immediate discomfort. I like to remind that majority of clients who choose to continue with treatments that trying not to feel doesn't make things go away; it just stores them right back in the body to be dealt with at a later time.

To help cleanse any released toxicity from your body after a treatment, I recommend Epsom salt baths, along with increased hydration.

Also, I personally am a big fan of mung bean dhal, made from small lentil-like legumes that have a wonderfully detoxifying effect (I picked up this wisdom from a gifted Ayurvedic practitioner).

How much MFR is too much?

In the world of bodywork, it's generally not recommended that people receive more than one spa massage in a day, or even in two days. The body can become sore and achy from the lactic acid produced from effleurage (sweeping) and petrissage (squeezing) of the muscles using oil or lotion and from having the direct pinpoint pressure on sore spots that are common practice in deep tissue massage.

It's possible, however, to receive an intensive series of MFR treatments (for instance, three times a day, three days in a row) because, as layers of fascial restriction are cleared, the holding patterns are opening and expanding and letting go of stored toxicity, allowing the blood to carry away those toxic byproducts.

In myofascial release the focus is not on individual muscles, because it's the whole-body fascial system that's being treated. During any session where stretching interrupts a holding pattern, the layers of holding under and around it also need to be addressed. The more time you allow to elapse between treatments, the more the old pattern of holding has a chance to settle back in as the elastin component returns to the position it "remembers". We want to establish new memories in your fascia.

So, to maintain the progress made in the session before, and move in the most expeditious way toward further release in the deeper fascial layers, I recommend scheduling MFR treatments close together—in some cases, even having several on the same day.

How soon after surgery or an injury is it safe to receive MFR?

The sooner, the better. You don't want the freeze response to continue. If the fascial restriction that occurs after surgery or an injury is allowed to persist, it will deprive the tissues of circulation. Without circulation, the wounded area doesn't receive oxygen, resulting in a condition known as hypoxia. The area will appear pale and feel cold to the touch, and this hypoxic condition will impair the healing process.

Because the work is done very gently, and in post-traumatic cases consists chiefly of traction on the extremities, the scar or injury doesn't need to be directly touched immediately after the event. MFR facilitates the rest-and-restore reaction of the parasympathetic nervous system, and clears a path for blood flow to the site.

In the days and weeks that follow, there can be more direct contact in the area of the wound to prevent keloid scarring and tissue derangement.

Remember my first MFR instructor, Tina? When she fractured her neck, she immediately called her team of MFR colleagues into the hospital room, and received gentle traction from them in the days after the accident. Her recovery was remarkable, and, seeing her, you would never guess she had once broken her neck.

You can go online to www.painreliefsanctuary.com/mfr-after-surgery/ or scan the QR code on the next page to see two X-rays of the same broken collarbone—the first taken just after the injury and the second taken following an MFR treatment. (This excerpt from a John Barnes brochure is used by permission.)

What happens if I start a series of MFR treatments and then decide to either take a break (because I have too much going on in my life) or stop (because it feels like I'm getting worse)?

As a myofascial specialist, I've seen this happen many times. If you back off, allowing other priorities of your life to interfere with you giving your body the treatment it needs, it can mean that you and your MFR therapist will need to travel the same ground over and over again.

I've done this myself as an MFR recipient, and have consequently found myself hanging out for too long in painful places of struggle in my body.

For you to benefit from all that MFR can offer, you need to know that it's not a passive experience, but one that calls for you to face your fears and keep peeling back the layers of the onion.

If you take a break, you can't make the kind of progress you can make if you stick with it for a period of time and receive treatments spaced closely together. There's no simple formula for calculating how long that period of time will be. It will have a lot to do with your commitment and willingness to feel and to heal.

The healing journey doesn't follow a straight line, and no two clients experience their treatment in the same way. Some breeze right through it, and for others it takes more time.

As you learn to tune in to your fascial voice and tune out the external stimuli bombarding you, you'll begin to shed the layers of internal holding that have been gripping you for a lifetime.

I know, because of my own experience and the hundreds of client experiences I've been witness to, that there's actual light at the end of all those fascial tunnels. As a client looks imploringly into my eyes, I can only hope that he'll hang in there and ultimately trust that his body is his partner, not his enemy.

Yet sometimes a client's belief that resolution should happen quickly, that her pain is somehow unique and unconquerable, or that she will spend money and have nothing to show for it is too strong. In such a case, I have to trust that there's a right time for everything—or a better client-therapist match for her out there somewhere—and follow my own advice to let go.

Chapter Fourteen
Fascia in the Future

As I've made my way through the slings and arrows of physical existence, all the fear, heartache, accidents, injuries, surgeries—even giving birth—have led me to seek help and have ultimately brought me to a better understanding of what works.

I'm grateful for the perspective that time can bring, as so often I didn't understand what good could possibly come from what I was going through. Much of what I've had to learn has been about fear and resistance.

What I've shared with you in these pages is about love and letting go. I've only lived perhaps half of my life, and I certainly don't pretend to know it all . . . I'm always looking forward to finding out what's next. But, for now, I'm sharing what I've learned so far.

I began my mission to spread the word about myofascial release in 2003. Through the subsequent years, I've come to realize just how challenging it is to put the whole subject of MFR into words. It's so much easier for me to communicate through touch.

However, with time and practice I've found words that enhance the understanding and experience of each client on my treatment table and each student in my classes—words that I repeat again and again. In this book, I've undertaken to write for a large readership what I've been saying to one class or one person at a time. Getting it all written down in one place is giving me great satisfaction.

I've learned that whoever needs me seems to somehow show up at my office. One particular person who found his way to me inspired me to write. He was so moved by what he was able to accomplish with MFR that he began to encourage me every time he came in for an appointment.

When I would speak the words I've found to describe the processes of MFR, he'd say, "You've got to write that down."

Or, "Where did you learn this?"

Or, "Everyone should know about this!"

So I began to write this book, starting out with just the informative bare bones. It was then that it began to dawn on me that it's been my challenges and life experiences that have brought me to the work I do and helped me to understand it so well.

It's my wish that, through revealing in this book some of those adventures and misadventures, I can help you to gain a more appreciative insight into your own life experiences and their effects.

My Speculations about Fascia

Light carries information. Does this mean that the fascial web is full of information? And, if so, what kind? This quote from Lynn McTaggart's *The Field* shows you one theory at which scientists have arrived and where they're going with it:

"Yasui, Pribram, Hameroff, and Hagan from the Department of physics at McGill University formulated a theory about the nature of human consciousness.

"According to the theory, microtubules and the membranes of dendrites represent the Internet of the body."

McTaggart goes on to say, "Microtubules help to marshal discordant energy and create global coherence of the waves of the body, in a process called Super Radiance."

"Once coherence was achieved the photons could travel all along the light pipes as if they were transparent. A phenomenon called Self-Induced Transparency." To me, this information from *The Field* indicates that we're capable of "turning on the lights" inside of us.

I find this theory exciting. There's a reason, then, why we use words like *glow* and *shine,* and phrases such as *lights up a room.* We all know people who can be described this way, and we've probably at times been described this way ourselves.

If fascia is fluid-filled and conducts light, let's speculate about those properties of fluid, light, vibration, and frequency. If those fluid-filled tubules vibrate, is that the mechanism by which we pick up on other people's energy and mood?

I've often wondered how fascia would be affected if one were to float in a pool of water heated to body temperature and infused with varying vibrational frequencies as well as with light moving through a spectrum of color. I don't mean a sensory deprivation tank. I'm speculating about something a little more intentional from a fascial perspective.

I'm also a practitioner of a form of bodywork whose originator, Harold Dull, experimented by performing Zen Shiatsu in the heated pools of Harbin Hot Springs in Middletown, California. This led him to create the now world-renowned practice of Watsu®, a sublime experience of floating in body-temperature water while the practitioner holds you and manipulates your limbs and all you have to do is let go. It's like returning to the womb. I would love to combine this modality with MFR and see where it might take us.

Could one learn to exert conscious control of one's fascia? Could one increase one's glow by the use of intention? Is dancing just one big unwinding of snarled fascia?

Also, what's happening with fascia during an orgasm? Does it grip and grip and grip until it releases and then is it lit up all throughout the body at once? Do we thwart orgasm in an effort to be quiet and regain our dignity? If we were to allow an unwinding of the orgasm, just how much noise and movement could occur? Is every orgasm an opportunity to unwind fascia?

Consider the old-fashioned term "nervous breakdown." What, exactly, does that entail?

Does a person just get to the point where he can't contain all that stored-up holding anymore and surrender to hysteria? Is the catatonic aftermath that sometimes results just an absence of tension, or has the holding overtaken everything?

And what role does fascia play in tremors? Are they evidence of an internal fight between letting go and keeping it together?

For restless leg syndrome, has anyone prescribed kicking? Imagine all the times you might have felt like kicking someone, but restrained yourself instead. Could a regular, hearty temper tantrum to empty out all of those withheld kicks provide the needed relief?

Knowing what we do about the fascial web and our connection to each other, can we speculate that people exchange information by emanating frequency and light? Might this be what we call intuition, telepathy, clairvoyance? Maybe ESP is not so extrasensory, after all.

When Are We Done?

The simple answer? Never. We're here on this earth having a physical experience. Every day of our life we're subject to gravity, strong emotions, sudden fearful noises, and other humans with their own agendas, each encounter presenting a fresh opportunity to clench.

By understanding your fascial web, you have a way to interrupt your holding patterns quickly, before long-term denial and resistance settle in and you become unconscious of their strangling grip.

In the expanding field of self-help, a great deal of focus is placed on the mind and spirit. In the field of fitness, there's equal focus on the appearance of the body as related to diet and exercise. With your new understanding of fascia, you can see that ignoring the mind and spirit doesn't work for the body—nor does punishing it with exercise that creates micro tears and hardens it to the point of inflexibility.

Feeling, movement, stretching, unwinding, calming the panic, and planned (safe) temper tantrums are your new tools for interrupting unconscious holding patterns and handling life as it happens.

You no longer need to try to guess which singular component needs adjustment, removal, or drugs. When discomfort visits you, you can first ask:

Where do I feel squeezed or pulled on from the inside?

What am I trying not to feel?

And, instead of gripping, release and soften. Loosening the grip of your mind and your fascia will allow your body to lead you back out into the great wide open.

Chapter Fifteen
Wrapping It Up

We are movement creatures. Remember—just because you don't *have* to move much in your life anymore doesn't mean that you don't need to. My focus is not on fitness, with its emphasis on appearance. I'm focused on wellness, with its emphasis on feeling. When you experience joy and ease of movement in your body, you raise the vibration of everyone around you no matter what your appearance is.

As many of us in the Baby Boomer generation approach our golden years, we're coming to a realization. We've spent a huge amount of time (and earned a great deal of money) using our heads. However, our bodies are now crying out for attention.

We're noticing how Western medicine has been offering us only prescriptions to dull the symptoms, and surgery to cut out the parts that hurt.

Many have voted with their feet by not returning to the doctor's office, and have instead gone searching for alternatives. We're learning that our health is as much a reflection of our thinking as it is a result of diet and exercise. And we're placing much new emphasis on the body chemistry in our fascia, produced by our thinking.

The body environment that Bruce Lipton describes is contained by a fascial web, and knowledge of the role played by this web provides a critical link that's been missing from our understanding of every area of health—body, mind, and spirit.

We can go to a transformational weekend seminar and have a breakthrough in our thinking that leads us to greater possibilities for happiness, but this gets clouded over by the physical pain of sitting in those chairs all weekend.

In the seminar, we might access the potential to create the life of our dreams, but our knees, back, and neck hurt, we develop a headache, and when we get home we can't spend much time at the computer manifesting that new life because using the mouse and keyboard makes our hands go numb.

We might solve a physical issue with surgery, then find that the resultant scarring interferes so much with our digestion, joint mobility, or physical ease that we can no longer enjoy the simple freedom of movement.

This book is not about technique, but truth. In these pages you've learned something about your body that will allow you much more say in your own well-being.

Wheatgrass, HGH, colon cleansing, crystal healing, vision questing, and organic, gluten-free, or non-GMO foods are all wonderful things, as are hiking, biking, swimming, yoga, Pilates, and gym membership . . . *and* you now have another piece to the healing puzzle that will give you enormous help in making sense of it all.

How lucky we are to live in a time when science has brought us fiber-optic cameras and video recording devices, so that we can see into the microscopic corners of the body and discover that . . . lo and behold . . . each and every one of us is made up of our own all-encompassing system of fiber optics.

My intent in writing this book has been to share my knowledge of what actually works in the prevention and treatment of pain, injury, and joint deterioration. You, having read it, now know the power you have to self-heal and to maintain your vitality.

I want to inspire my readers to regard their body as I regard my own: with appreciation for its light-bearing fascia. By sharing what works, I want to start a new movement toward improved health. I dream of a widespread revolution in our understanding and treatment of the human body. I hope that my own fascination with fascia can inspire . . . a fascia nation!

Epilogue

After reading the final draft of this book, my dear sister, Bonnie, said, "Okay. You've sold me. Where do I start?" Somehow it hadn't yet occurred to me that my readers might want to know how to sign up for this particular brand of treatment. I'm grateful that my sister brought this to my attention prior to publication, so that I can be quite clear about how my readers can visit us at our Ojai Healing Movement Sanctuary to take a taste, try a few bites, or enjoy a full meal of what we're cooking. I predict that you'll realize right away that total immersion is the best way to go.

Here in Ojai, we host workshops that include True Body™ classes and myofascial release treatments. Whether you visit us in our beautiful California resort town (search "Ojai, California" on Wikipedia to view this page) . . .

. . . or invite us to come teach in your own distant city, we'll provide you with a safe container for letting go to achieve long-lasting, authentic healing.

If you consider yourself a potential MFR practitioner, your first step is to visit our website, www.ohmsanctuary.com. After having your own initial True Body™ experience, if your heart tells you that you'd like to learn the unique combination of skills that I teach, I encourage you to enroll in our practitioner training.

If you're already a nurse, OT, PT, ST, LMT, EMT, physician, minister, chiropractor, cosmetologist, esthetician, or otherwise "licensed to touch," you've already qualified yourself to begin your training in myofascial release.

About the Author

Ronelle Wood received her Master of Science in Speech/Language Pathology from California State University, Sacramento, in 1988; her Massage Therapy License from Santa Barbara School of Massage in 1994; and her Myofascial Release Technique training from John F. Barnes, PT, in 2003-2008. In 2007 she was certified by Harold Dull as a Level 3 Watsu® Practitioner.

She worked in Ventura, California, as a myofascial release specialist at Restorative Exercise Institute from 2007-2009 and, with her partner, Joe Cocke, has co-owned and co-operated Ojai Healing Movement/Sanctuary (www.ohmsanctuary.com) in Ojai, California, from 2010 to the present.

Ronelle says that, following an injury, she went in search of what works. In *Touching Light* she describes "the things I found that brought me authentic, long-term healing." She adds, "Now I get to pay it forward."

Her goal is to imbue her clients with a love of movement and, through facilitating myofascial release and alignment, empower them to maintain lifelong health and independence.

Ronelle's loves include her daughter and son, Genevieve and Alex; her partner, Joe, and his daughter, SammiJo; and living in Ojai. Her favorite pastimes are singing, beading, walking, playing table tennis, and putting together jigsaw puzzles.

Made in the USA
San Bernardino, CA
13 September 2016